Integrative Dermatology

Reena N. Rupani • Peter A. Lio
Editors

Integrative Dermatology

Practical Applications in Acne and Rosacea

Springer

Editors
Reena N. Rupani
Department of Dermatology
Icahn School of Medicine at Mount Sinai
New York, NY
USA

Peter A. Lio
Department of Dermatology & Pediatrics, Northwestern University Feinberg School of Medicine
Chicago, IL
USA

ISBN 978-3-030-58953-0 ISBN 978-3-030-58954-7 (eBook)
https://doi.org/10.1007/978-3-030-58954-7

This Springer imprint is published by the registered company Springer Nature Switzerland AG
The registered company address is: Gewerbestrasse 11, 6330 Cham, Switzerland

For Rai and Lilia, but most of all, my Rishi

–Reena N. Rupani

To my children, Nathan and Elena, for always keeping me on my toes!

–Peter A. Lio

Preface

The Integrative Health movement continues to grow and develop in the United States and throughout the world. The National Institutes of Health/National Center for Complementary and Integrative Health notes that more than 30% of adults and some 12% of children utilize healing approaches outside of conventional medicine [1]. Driven partly by patients seeking holistic and personalized care, and partly by clinicians striving to incorporate mental, emotional, functional, spiritual, social, and community aspects of healing in step with conventional drug development pathways, there is undoubtedly an appeal of Integrative Health that enhances the connection between patient and provider—somewhat of a harkening back to the village doctor who knew all of the individual stories.

The vast majority of our modern medicines stem from simpler and more natural beginnings, such as plants used by various world traditions for generations. Integrative Health offers the chance to look to these simpler, more elemental therapies for new ideas and approaches that, ironically, may one day be quite mainstream and may serve as valuable adjuncts to current allopathic standards of care.

As clinicians, we are sometimes painfully aware of the limitations of conventional medicine. Indeed, as Celsius once quipped: "*Satius est enim anceps auxilium experiri quam nullum*" or "It is better to try a doubtful remedy than none at all" [2]. Despite the best and most robust evidence, there are often scenarios where the data is lacking or the patient simply has not responded to what evidence-based literature deems best; there may be a need for adjunctive botanical or behavioral therapy to help mitigate adverse effects of standard care; perhaps the real or perceived side effects of a group of treatment options actually outweigh their potential therapeutic benefit, prompting a change of course; or, more fundamentally, a patient may benefit from a sense of agency which can come with addressing diet, discussing specific stressors, or even highlighting the simple concept of sleep hygiene.

In dermatology, we feel this equally or perhaps even more acutely than other medical fields—we are mandated to treat a number of ill-defined and chronic inflammatory conditions, most of which have little chance of cure. We look forward to exploring the concept and applications of Integrative Dermatology with you, our colleagues and community, and hope that at the very least, the conversation is stimulating.

References

1. https://nccih.nih.gov/health/integrative-health
2. Spivack BS. A. C. Celsus: Roman medicus. J Hist Med Allied Sci. 1991;46:143–57.

New York, NY, USA — Reena N. Rupani
Chicago, IL, USA — Peter A. Lio

Introduction

> Integrative dermatology is as much a philosophy as it is a method; it looks to reverse causal factors rather than just stop symptoms. [1]

What better dermatologic illness to start the discussion of nutrition, stress, lifestyle, and role of supplements and botanical ingredients than acne? In this volume we focus on the treatment of Acneiform disorders, specifically acne vulgaris, with discussion too of rosacea. Assuming a target audience of skilled dermatologists, internists, pediatricians, and family medicine providers, standard medical approaches to acne are considered the foundation upon which our discussion of integrative therapies will rest.

The first part of the book (Chaps. 1, 2, and 3) begins with a discussion of the skin and gut microbiome as well as the use of oral supplements, including pre/probiotics, vitamins, minerals, and botanical ingredients.

Chapters 4 and 5 will consider non-prescription topical botanical therapies and essential oils.

In Chap. 6, the somewhat novel (to dermatology) concept of Apitherapy is introduced, with consideration of naturally derived bee products, such as honey, propolis, and bee venom, and potential role in acne/rosacea therapy.

Chapter 7 delves deeply into the hot topic of diet and acne/rosacea, including not only dairy and glycemic load, but also specific diet plans (Mediterranean, plant-based, low histamine) as well as anti-inflammatory dietary approaches.

Chapter 8 discusses the important role of stress in acne and rosacea, and specific mind–body interventions that can significantly improve patient outcomes.

For those who are unfamiliar with the field of functional medicine, Chap. 9 will introduce the core areas of Assimilation/Gastrointestinal, Immune, Energy, Detoxification, Cardiovascular/Lymphatic, Hormones/Neurotransmitter, and Musculoskeletal/Cellular Structure, and the connection between each of these areas and acne/rosacea.

The millenia-old system of Ayurvedic medicine, which originates from and is still practiced regularly in the Indian subcontinent, is defined in Chap. 10, with specific relevance to acne/rosacea therapy.

By turn, Chap. 11 explores traditional Chinese medicine as a complete healing system, and how practitioners characterize and treat acne/rosacea within this framework.

Finally, Chap. 12 concludes with an introduction to homeopathy, a more than 200-year-old healing system based on the "law of similars," with specific focus on the treatment of acne and rosacea.

We hope that this book is informative and instructive, and helps to generate ideas for future applications and research.

Reference

1. Norman RA, Shenefelt PD, Rupani RN. Integrative dermatology. Oxford: Oxford University Press; 2014.

New York, NY, USA — Reena N. Rupani
Chicago, IL, USA — Peter A. Lio

Contents

Contributors

Hilary E. Baldwin, MD Department of Dermatology, Rutgers Robert Wood Johnson, Piscataway, NJ, USA

Keira L. Barr, MD Resilient Health Institute, Gig Harbor, WA, USA

Valeria De Bedout, MD Dr. Phillip Frost Department of Dermatology and Cutaneous Surgery, University of Miami Miller School of Medicine, Miami, FL, USA

Marissa Ceresnie, DO Nova Southeastern University College of Osteopathic Medicine, Davie, FL, USA

Neha Chandan, MD, MPH Department of Dermatology, University of Illinois Hospital & Health Sciences System, Chicago, IL, USA

Sara Dill, MD Luminous Dermatology, Santa Barbara, CA, USA

Jacquelyn Dosal, MD Department of Dermatology, Skin Associates of South Florida, Coral Gables, FL, USA

Shala Fardin, MD Southern Marin Dermatology, Sausalito, CA, USA

Jessica Maria May Franklin, DO Edward Via College of Osteopathic Medicine – Virginia Campus, Blacksburg, VA, USA

Matthew Goldberg, MD Department of Dermatology, Icahn School of Medicine at Mount Sinai, New York, NY, USA

Joanna N. Hooten, MD Clara Dermatology, Cary, NC, USA

Michelle Jeffries, DO, PLLC Private Practice, Scottsdale, AZ, USA

Mamta Jhaveri, MD, MS, FAAD Johns Hopkins Dermatology, Washington, DC, USA

Jonette Keri, MD, PhD Philip Frost Department of Dermatology and Cutaneous Surgery, University of Miami, Miller School of Medicine, Miami, FL, USA

Marit K. Kreidel, MD Department of Dermatology, Kaiser Permanente, Irvine, CA, USA

Adriana Leite, MD Department of Dermatology, All Beauty Company, São Paulo, Brazil

Peter A. Lio, MD Department of Dermatology & Pediatrics, Northwestern University Feinberg School of Medicine, Chicago, IL, USA

Justin W. Marson, MD Internal Medicine, University of California, Irvine Medical Center, Orange, CA, USA

Anna J. Nichols, MD, PhD Clinical Trials Unit, High Risk Skin Cancer Clinic, Dr. Phillip Frost Department of Dermatology and Cutaneous Surgery, University of Miami Miller School of Medicine, Sylvester Comprehensive Cancer Center, Miami, FL, USA

Lawrence Chukwudi Nwabudike, MBBS, MRCP(UK), PhD Department of Outpatient Dermatology, N. Paulescu National Institute of Diabetes, Bucharest, Romania

Aunna Pourang, MD Department of Dermatology, University of California – Davis, Sacramento, CA, USA

Reena N. Rupani, MD Department of Dermatology, Icahn School of Medicine at Mount Sinai, New York, NY, USA

Lauren Schwartzberg, BS, OMS-II New York Institute of Technology College of Osteopathic Medicine, Old Westbury, NY, USA

Raja K. Sivamani, MD, MS, AP Department of Dermatology, University of California – Davis, Sacramento, CA, USA

Michal Solomon, MD Department of Dermatology, Sheba Medical Center, Ramat Gan, Israel

Carol Ann Soutor, MD Department of Dermatology, University of Minnesota Medical Center, Minneapolis, MN, USA

Valori Treloar, MD, CNS Integrative Dermatology, Newton, MA, USA

Abbreviations

Acne-QoL	acne-specific quality-of-life
AhR	Aryl hydrocarbon receptor
AMPs	Antimicrobial peptides
AV	Acne vulgaris
BCMO1	Beta carotene mono oxidase 1
BPH	Benign prostatic hypertrophy
BPO	Benzoyl peroxide
CAM	Complementary alternative medicine
CBD	Cannabinoid
CDC	Centers for Disease Control and Prevention
CoNS	Coagulase-negative staphylococcus
COX-2	Cyclooxygenase 2
CRH	Corticotropin-releasing hormone
CRP	C-reactive protein
DAO	Diamine oxidase
DHEA	Dehydroepiandrosterone
DIM	Diindolylmethane
EC	Epicatechin
ECG	Epicatechin-3-gallate
ECS	Endocannabinoid systems
EG	Epigallocatechin
EGCG	Epigallocatechin-3-gallate
EGFR	Epidermal growth factor receptor
EMA	European Medicines Agency
FFA	Free fatty acids
FODMAP	Fermentable oligosaccharides, disaccharides, monosaccharides, and polyols

FOX01	Forkhead box transcription factor/forkhead box 01
GAGS	Global Acne Grading System
GC	German chamomile
GL	Glycemic load
GTP	Phenolic fraction of green tea
H2O2	Hydrogen peroxide
HIF-1	Hypoxia-inducible factor-1
HMO	Human milk oligosaccharides
I3C	Indole-3-carbinol
ICAM-1	Intercellular cell adhesion molecule-1
IGA	Investigator Global Assessment
IGA-RSS	Investigator Global Assessment of Rosacea Severity Score
IGF-1	Insulin-like growth factor-1
IL	Insulinemic load
IL-1	Interleukin-1
IL-1A	Interleukin-1 alpha
IL-1B	Interleukin-1 beta
IL-1β	Interleukin 1β
IL-6	Interleukin-6
LDC-C	Low-density lipoprotein cholesterol
LPS	Ipopolysaccharides
LTF	Lost to follow-up
MAPK	Mitogen-activated protein kinases
MIC	Minimum inhibitory concentration
MRSA	Methicillin-resistant Staphylococcus aureus
mTOR1	Mechanistic target of rapamycin complex 1
mTORC1	Mammalian target of rapamycin complex
NAD	Nicotinamide adenine dinucleotide
NETs	Neutrophil extracellular traps
NFkB	Nuclear factor kappa B
OR	Odds ratio
PBV	Purified bee venom
PCOS	Polycystic ovarian syndrome
PI3K-AKT	Phosphoinositol-3-kinase – protein kinase B
PMNs	Polymorphonuclear neutrophils
PMS	Premenstrual syndrome

PRRs	Pattern recognition receptors
PS	Phytosphingosine
PSMs	Phenol-soluble modulins
PTAC	20% propolis tree extract, 3% tree tea oil, and 10% aloe vera leaf juice
PVL	Panton–Valentine leucocidin
ROS	Reactive oxygen species
RR	Relative risk
SCFAs	Short-chain fatty acids
SIBO	Small intestine bacterial overgrowth
TCM	Traditional Chinese medicine
TEWL	Transepidermal water loss
TLR	Toll-like receptor
TNF	Tumor necrosis factor
TRP	Transient receptor potential
TRPA1	Transient receptor potential ankyrin-1
TRPV	Transient receptor potential vanilloid channels (TRPV1-6)
TRPV1	Transient receptor potential vanilloid receptor 1
TTO	Tea tree oil
VAC	*Vitex agnus castus*
VCAM-1	Vascular cell adhesion protein-1
VEGF	Vascular endothelial growth factor

Chapter 1
The Microbiome, Probiotics, and Prebiotics

Shala Fardin and Jonette Keri

Microbiome Overview

A relatively new and rapidly expanding field of research involves characterizing the human microbiome. The microgenome refers to the genetics of the microbiota, while microbiota are all the microbial cells of a region or body. The microbiome includes microbiota plus their genetic material, while the metagenome includes the total genetic material of microbes inhabiting our bodies and is much more variable than human genome [1]. The macrobiome refers to the ecological health and biodiversity of the surrounding environment [2]. It is estimated that 100 trillion (10^{14}) microorganisms live in and on our bodies—tenfold the number of human cells [3, 4]. In a square centimeter of the skin, it is estimated that over 100 distinct species comprise a total of one million bacteria, and there are up to one billion microorganisms colonizing this space when factoring in fungi, mites, and viruses [4–6]. Given

S. Fardin
Southern Marin Dermatology, Sausalito, CA, USA

J. Keri (✉)
Philip Frost Department of Dermatology and Cutaneous Surgery, University of Miami, Miller School of Medicine, Miami, FL, USA
e-mail: JKeri@med.miami.edu

R. N. Rupani, P. A. Lio (eds.), *Integrative Dermatology*,
https://doi.org/10.1007/978-3-030-58954-7_1

each species has a unique genotype comprised of thousands of genes, it is humbling to comprehend that the genetic content of the microbiome far exceeds that of our human genome [7].

There is a large degree of interpersonal diversity in the gut and skin microbiomes [1]. Twin studies have shown that the microbiome is influenced by genetics, skin pigmentation, age, and shared environment; twins also show a high degree of interpersonal diversity as well [1, 2, 8]. Variability in microenvironments for different sites on the skin and great variability in external treatment of the skin by different individuals makes it difficult to establish clear relationships between the presence of specific organisms and skin functions [9]. However, many microbial genes are preserved among all individuals, and thus it has been proposed that a healthy "functional core" exists, resulting from the functional benefit of a given microbiome in a particular habitat which provides essential metabolic and other molecular functions, rather than a "healthy microbiome" defined by taxonomy [1]. A well-functioning microbiome must be resilient to stressors and disruption [1]. A change in the diversity of microbiota, such as increased diversity of a normally restricted microbiome habitat or decreased diversity in one that is typically highly diverse, is associated with disease [10].

With regard to acne and rosacea, the gut microbiome and skin microbiome have the most well-studied interactions. In the following sections, we will highlight the structure and function of the gut and skin microbiomes in their normal and diseased contexts and review the microbiome changes in each disease state. Finally, we will review therapeutic options such as prebiotics and probiotics.

Gut Microbiome

Most extensively studied to date is the gut microbiome. The microbiome of the human gastrointestinal system is similar to the skin, as there are also regional differences. The oral cavity, stomach, small intestine, and large intestine all have distinct microbiomes. Interestingly, the skin and the gut have the same dominant phyla but in different proportions [11]. The human gut contains nearly 10 trillion bacterial cells and over 2000 different species [4]. Lifestyle choices such as mode of birth delivery and feeding modality, improved sanitation, introduction of antibiotics and vaccines, a Western diet, environment, genetic predispositions, and consumption of artificial nutrients greatly impact the gut microbiota [4, 9].

In the gut, antibiotics were found to cause not only a transient loss in bacterial diversity but also a long-term loss of microbiome members beyond the direct antibiotic targets [6]. These changes in the composition of the microbiome, even after the bacterial density has been restored, facilitate colonization by pathogens such as vancomycin-resistant *Enterococcus* [6]. It can take years until the normal microbiota recovers, and thus it is essential as dermatologists to be aware of the impact of short- and long-term antibiotic use in our patients [9].

Gut symbionts such as *Bacteroides*, *Parabacteroides*, *Clostridium*, *Lactobacillus*, *Bifidobacterium*, and *Faecalibacterium prausnitzii* provide several determinants of a healthy microbiome, and once established, these are the main producers of short-chain fatty acids (SCFAs), an important source of energy from non-digestible carbohydrates [1]. SCFAs are immunomodulatory, inhibiting common pathogens, and potentially having tumor-suppressive properties [1]. Those gut microbiota strongly affect adaptive immunity, and the development and homeostasis of the host is well-known. For example, *Bacteroides fragilis*, a common commensal, activates regulatory T cells and stimulates production of anti-inflammatory cytokines, primarily interleukin (IL)-10 [6].

Diet represents a strong selective pressure on the microbiome, and breastfeeding favors certain microbial clades from the initial microbiota which may have assembled at random. Human milk oligosaccharides (HMO) can be used as the sole carbon source by only a handful of *Bifidobacterium* and *Bacteroides* species [1]. This functional profile is established early on in life and remains stable thereafter. The gut microbiota functions include glycosaminoglycan biodegradation, production of SCFAs, enrichment for specific lipopolysaccharides, and the production of vitamins and essential amino acids [1].

Disturbances in gut microbiota have been shown to contribute to diseases of immune dysregulation [6]. Germ-free mice exhibit defective development of gut-associated lymphoid tissue and mesenteric lymph nodes, reduced epithelial expression of immune molecules, and improper T-cell differentiation [6]. Dysbiosis is a disruption of the normal microbial composition leading to abnormal host–microbe interactions. An imbalance of oral and gastrointestinal microorganisms has been linked to various systemic diseases such as obesity, inflammatory bowel disease, multiple sclerosis, types 1 and 2 diabetes, cancer, autoimmune diseases such as rheumatoid arthritis, allergies, and asthma [1, 9, 12]. Studies suggest composition of the gut microbiome can even affect the efficacy of cancer immunotherapies [12]. The impact of gut microorganisms on acne and rosacea is still being elucidated.

The discussion of this section will deal mainly with the gut microbiome and the relationship to the skin. Amazingly, the intestinal microbiome can contribute to skin allostasis after a stressor. Gut bacteria can improve a disturbed barrier of the skin. Administration of *Lactobacillus helveticus* decreased transepidermal water loss (TEWL) and the dermatitis induced by sodium dodecyl sulfate [13]. Another lactobacillus, *Lactobacillus paracasei* CNCM I-2116, has also been shown to improve the skin barrier and decrease signs of inflammation of the skin [14–16]. In addition, wounded mice had accelerated wound healing after eating *Lactobacillus reuteri* [17].

Acne and the Gut Microbiome

One theory supporting cross talk between the intestinal commensal bacterial and inflammatory mediators of acne pathogenesis suggests that diets with a high glycemic load, which have been implicated in acne, lead to increased insulin and insulin-like growth factor-1 (IGF-1). These increases in insulin and IGF-1 then lead to increased expression of the metabolic forkhead box transcription factor (FOX01). The FOXO1 goes on to trigger mammalian target of rapamycin complex (mTORC1) which then mediates acne lesion formation by sebaceous gland hyperplasia, lipogenesis, and hyperplasia of infundibular keratinocytes [18].

The above theory was evaluated in patients who were supplemented with *Lactobacillus rhamnosus* SP1. The study by Fabbrocini et al. was of 20 adults (14 women and 6 men) who were treated for 12 weeks with the above *Lactobacillus* probiotic [19]. The patients had skin biopsies before and at the end of the 12 weeks' treatment period and were found to have a significant reduction in IGF-1 and FOXO1 gene expression. In addition, the patients in the probiotic groups were rated to be improved/markedly improved versus placebo (adjusted odds ratio 28.4). A second theory supporting acne and GI dysfunction includes a role for the brain in addition to the gut and a hypothesis that the gut–brain–skin axis suggests that upregulation of substance P is seen in both acne and intestinal dysbiosis [18]. A third theory suggests that hypochlorhydria is associated with acne, and, with low levels of acid in the small intestine, there may be some small intestinal bacterial overgrowth which then leads ultimately to systemic inflammation [18, 20].

Gut Microbiota in Acne Patients

Studies to define the gut microbiome date back to the 1930s [21] and then move into recent times. In two recent studies, the gut microbiota has been evaluated in acne patients versus healthy controls [22, 23]. Deng et al. examined 43 Chinese treatment-naïve acne patients and compared their microbiota to healthy controls [22]. Stool samples were collected and analyzed, and acne patients had less diversity of their gut flora. The patients with acne also had specific differences including more of the phylum *Bacteroidetes* and less of the

Firmicutes. The acne patients also had less of four other groups including *Clostridia*, *Clostridiales*, *Lachnospiraceae*, and *Ruminococcaceae* genera.

In a second study of 31 patients and matched controls—who had not used systemic antibiotics, retinoids, corticosteroids, or immunosuppressants in the last 2 months—stool samples were obtained and analyzed [23]. There was a significant difference between the two groups with respect to gut microbiota. *Actinobacteria* was reduced in the acne patients (0.89%) versus control (2.84%, $P = 0.004$), and *Proteobacteria* was increased in acne patients (8.35%) versus controls (7.01%, $p = 0.031$). Acne patients, at the genus level, had less *Bifidobacterium*, *Butyricicoccus*, *Coprobacillus*, *Lactobacillus*, and *Allobaculum*. There is speculation that such changes in the microbiota lead to an environment that is more inflammatory and may have far-reaching effects from the gut to the skin and an overall systemic inflammatory state.

Studies of Interventions that May Help Acne Patients

Both oral and topical interventions have been studied with respect to acne patients. An early study looking at oral supplementation of patients with freeze-dried *L. acidophilus* and *Bifidobacterium* as an addition to therapy showed patients with better clinical outcomes and with better tolerance to antibiotics [24]. Later studies again have shown that probiotics with antibiotics give a more rapid improvement [25]. In a study from 2013 [26], when women were given minocycline alone, probiotics alone, or both minocycline and probiotics, all groups improved, with the combination group doing the best. The probiotic used in this study consisted of *Lactobacillus acidophilus*, *Lactobacillus delbrueckii* subspecies *bulgaricus*, and *Bifidobacterium bifidum*.

Plant extracts that may influence the gut microbiome and then help treat acne were reviewed by Clark et al. [27]. Studies which were randomized, controlled trials are reviewed here. Green tea extract (1500 mg of decaffeinated extract) was shown to decrease acne lesion counts in women ages 25–45 years old [28]. Gugulipid, which has antimicrobial as well as anti-inflammatory properties, was compared to 500 mg of tetracycline and found to be slightly more effective, and patients felt the skin to be less oily [29]. Berberine, a substance used in traditional Chinese medicine, which is believed to help with insulin resistance, was shown to be as effective as minocycline in patients with acne [30].

Rosacea and the Gut Microbiome

Patients with rosacea have been found to have more gastrointestinal illnesses. The increase in incidence in *Helicobacter pylori*, small intestine bacterial overgrowth (SIBO), inflammatory bowel disease, celiac disease, and irritable bowel syndrome have all been documented in the literature [31, 32]. Treatment of *H. pylori* and SIBO with antibiotics has been shown to improve rosacea in patients, although the connection between *H. pylori* and rosacea remains controversial. Interestingly, treatment of SIBO with a single 10-day course of rifaximin had a sustained remission of disease up to 3 years in some patients [33].

Since there is an association between GI illness and rosacea, the role of the gut microbiome in these illnesses is an area of interest. Recommendation for increased prebiotics for the rosacea patient makes sense, as this would promote a healthy gut microbiome. In fact, one case report using a high-fiber diet showed an improvement in rosacea, thought to be a reflection of shorter gut transit time [34].

Examination of the stool from Korean rosacea patients versus controls also found no statistical difference in the microbial diversity [35]. The patients had a similar amount of bacteria, but of a different composition. There were differences in the overall percentages of the unique genera. For example, *Acidaminococcus* and *Megasphaera* were significantly increased in rosacea patients, and *Methanobrevibacter* were significantly less abundant in rosacea patients. The influence of each of these bacteria on the gut–skin connection has yet to be determined [35].

There is less data with respect to which pre- and probiotic treatments will help treat rosacea. A single case report of scalp rosacea responded to low-dose doxycycline and a probiotic of an 8-week course of doxycycline 40 mg once a day and probiotic therapy twice a day (*Bifidobacterium breve* BR03, *Lactobacillus salivarius* LS01) [36]. However, the gastrointestinal system's microbiome remains a target of interest in this condition, and the agents which help in the treatment of acne may also be beneficial for the treatment of rosacea.

Skin Microbiome

Formation of the Skin Microbiome

Microbiome interactions may begin as early as in utero via the placenta, which has a rich microbiome. The skin, however, is primarily colonized by bacteria at birth by either the mother's vaginal flora (for vaginal deliveries) or by maternal skin flora (for cesarian sections), starting at very low density across the body [6, 37]. Lactobacilli dominate in neonatal skin versus propionibacteria in the mother [2]. *Bacillus*, *Clostridia*, and *Actinobacteria* are the most frequent classes found in infant skin [6]. Skin colonization by commensal skin microorganisms continues during breastfeeding [38]. Microorganisms from the environment also begin to colonize the skin, scalp, perigenital, and perioral areas such that, by adulthood, a final state of equilibrium is achieved with a highly diverse commensal/mutualistic microbiota that is unique at genus level for each individual [38].

Infants and children showed greater diversity than adults, and more than half of the bacterial sequences were either *Streptococcus*, *Staphylococcus*, *Propionibacterium*, *Prevotella*, or *Corynebacterium* [39]. Children's microbiomes in specific body habitats differ globally from the same sites in adults in terms of bacterial composition [6]. A continuous, gradual shift in the most dominant members of the skin microbiome from 3 weeks of age to adulthood occurs, with *Streptococcus* species becoming less dominant as *Propionibacterium* species increases [39].

The skin develops distinctive skin habitats that evolve with onset of puberty, aging, and environmental exposures [6]. During puberty, skin microbiota begin to be dominated by lipophilic bacteria, which reflect sexual maturation and is associated with increase in activity of hormone-stimulated sebaceous glands [8]. On adult skin, *Propionibacterium*, *Staphylococcus*, and *Streptococcus* comprise more than 60% of the total skin microbiome [39].

Composition of the Skin Microbiome

As stated previously, the composition of a "healthy microbiome" seen in the absence of any overt disease is difficult to fully characterize, as there is no ideal set of specific skin microbiota, but rather a functional ideal that can be created by many different microorganisms [1].

Microbiota of skin can be transient or resident, the latter being commensal skin microbiota that are in homeostasis with the host [5]. Considering that the skin is cool, dry, slightly acidic overall, and constantly shedding, the microbiome must be specially adapted to coexist with host cells despite various host antimicrobial defenses [4, 37, 40].

Bacteria are not uniformly distributed in the stratum corneum: the highest density is the surface layers, and very few bacteria exist near the stratum granulosum [5]. Microbes have been shown to extend down follicles and glands and into the dermal and fat component [5, 37]. The diversity of microbes of the skin stays relatively stable over time in a given individual [9].

The diversity and abundance of microbial flora depends on the topographical regions of the body that have distinctive characteristics (pH, moisture, salinity, sebum content) as well as genotype, age, gender, ethnicity, occupation, lifestyle, geographical location, hygiene, use of medications or antibiotics, cosmetics use, physiological injury, and even psychological anxiety [5, 9, 38, 40–42]. Endocrine and metabolic changes within the cutaneous microenvironments can directly impact the metabolic requirements and pathogenicity of various skin microorganisms [38].

Gender differences in skin microbiota may be due to variations in hormone production, sweat rate, sebum production, surface pH, skin thickness, hair growth, and cosmetics use.

There are many components of skin that shape a given local skin microbiome habitat. There is a distinct microbial community at the sebum-rich pilosebaceous unit; these microbes, like *Cutibacterium acnes* (formerly *Propionibacterium acnes*), can survive in this anoxic, lipid-rich environment by producing free fatty acids from sebum [37, 43]. Sebaceous glands constitutively express several antimicrobial peptides (AMPs) that are specific to multicellular organisms, such as cathelicidin, β-defensins, and antimicrobial histones, to help regulate microbial colonization [37].

Beyond these intrinsic components of the skin, external factors and individual behaviors create constant shifts and alterations of skin surfaces based on whether the skin is exposed or occluded, the degree of detergent or biocide use, the application of topicals and cosmetic products, occupational exposures, and the geography and composition of the home environment [37].

Topographical Variation in Skin Microbiome

Skin microbial composition is highly heterogeneous, with a great deal of variation among individuals and within a person, depending on the local microenvironment of a specific body site [2]. These site-based variations in microbes imply that no distinct "healthy microbiome" taxonomical community can be applied to the skin as a whole [37]. In addition, compared with the gut and oral microbiomes, the microbiome of the skin has the greatest variability over time [1].

The box lists the four predominant phyla and their relative percentage of composition of the total skin bacterial commensals [37, 40, 44]. Interestingly, the more highly culturable organisms *S. epidermidis* and *C. acnes* are commonly thought to be dominant bacteria residing on the skin, but they consisted of <5% of the microbiota captured by DNA extraction techniques [45].

Skin Microbiome Composition

Actinobacteria **(52%)**

- Gram-positive, aerobic, e.g., *Propionibacterium*, *Corynebacterium*, *Micrococcus*, *Brevibacterium*

Firmicutes **(24%)**

- Gram-positive, e.g., *Staphylococcus*, *Bacillus*, *Enterococcus*, *Gemella*, *Eubacterium*

Proteobacteria **(17%)**

- Gram-negative, *Enterobacteriaceae* and non-fermentative baccilli; *Pseudomonas*, *Stenotrophomonas*, *Acidovorax*, *Bradyrhizobium*, *Neisseria*, *Serratia*, *Methylobacterium*, *Sphingobium*, *Diaphorobacter*, *Enhydrobacter*

Bacteroidetes **(7%)**

- Gram-negative, *Bacteroides fragilis*, *Flavobacteriales*

In general, there are three broad cutaneous microenvironment types with their own characteristic microbial communities. Sebaceous gland-rich skin such as the forehead, external auditory canal, manubrium, retroauricular crease, and back harbor *Propionibacteria*, *Staphylococcus* species, and *Malassezia* predominantly [5, 8, 40, 42]. Moist areas, such as the toe web space, intergluteal cleft and axilla, inner elbow, and back of the knee, have abundant *Corynebacterium* species and also harbor gram-negative bacilli and *Staphylococcus* species [40, 42]. Moist areas are typically more stable, whereas dry environments have more change in composition [33]. Drier and more temperature-variable areas such as buttocks, forearms, and parts of the hands and legs have the most diversity, a greater prevalence of gram-negatives such as *β-proteobacteria* and *Flavobacteriales*, but the lowest colonization in absolute numbers [5, 40, 42]. *Proteobacteria* were previously thought to rarely colonize the skin and only as gastrointestinal contaminants, but are now clearly a significant part of the skin microbiome [6, 10, 44].

Other resident microorganisms present on the skin include viruses and eukaryotes, such as fungi, protozoa, and arthropods. *Malassezia globosa* (formerly *Pityrosporum ovale*), *Malassezia restricta*, and *Malassezia sympodialis* are the most frequent fungal isolates; they are lipophilic and frequently associated with sebum-rich areas of the skin [9]. *Candida albicans* and *Saccharomyces* are common yeasts that are pervasive on healthy skin [1, 9].

Lesser known skin microorganisms include protozoa, such as *Blastocystis*, and eukaryotes of the phylum Arthropoda, which include *Demodex* mites [1]. *Demodex* favor sebaceous skin—*Demodex folliculorum* is found in hair follicles in clusters with other mites of the same species, while *Demodex brevis* is a smaller mite and resides alone in sebaceous glands or meibomian glands of the eyelid rim [9].

The skin virome is least well-known, especially for RNA viruses. There does appear to be a high diversity of DNA viruses on human skin, but it is not yet clear if these are part of the skin microbiota or if they involve some mutual benefit to the host such as antimicrobial activity [9, 46]. A combination of stand-alone viruses and helper viruses has been detected in the follicular microbiome, suggesting that some mutualistic relationships may be critical to their colonization of the skin [47]. The virome is primarily comprised of bacteriophages, which provide an additional means of horizontal gene transfer among otherwise distantly related bacteria and are known to be present in *Staphylococcus*, *Pseudomonas*, and *Propionibacterium* species [1, 46].

Function of the Skin Microbiome

As the largest human organ, the skin provides a barrier to the outside world and to the macrobiome while also playing an important role in adapting our bodies to changing environments. Keratinocytes have been shown to function as an independent steroidogenic organ with the capacity to produce a wide variety of hormones, neurotransmitters, and cytokines that can potentially influence our physiology and possibly even our emotions [2]. Microbial–host interactions play an integral role in the maturation and homeostatic regulation of keratinocytes and host immune networks, with systemic implications for our overall health and well-being [2].

The skin microbiome has several key functions. Commensal bacteria help protect us from infection and invasion of pathogens by physically occupying space, competing for nutrients, and producing bacteria-specific AMPs called bacteriocins, which function to suppress competitor species [37]. In addition, the skin microbiome plays a critical role in the education and priming of adaptive immunity and in promoting host innate immunity [37].

Colonization of the skin during early neonatal life is essential for establishing adapted immune responses and tolerance to commensal microorganisms [38]. Early occupation of the skin by specific microbes triggers local activation of the host immune system in ways unique to infancy. For example, colonization by *Staphylococcus epidermidis* is associated with induction of *S. epidermidis*-specific T regulatory cells in neonatal, but not adult, skin [39]. These highly activated regulatory T cells abruptly flow into the neonatal skin, resulting in T-cell inhibition and tolerance to these commensals [38].

Commensal microbes epigenetically prime antigen-presenting cells to inform adaptive immunity, promoting self-tolerance and tolerance of commensal microbes via induction of regulatory T cells at steady state while also affecting host innate immunity. The skin's immune system can control the microbiome as well, reacting and modifying in response to a changing microbiota. Many skin microbes produce short-chain fatty acids as their metabolic waste, and thus the quantity of SCFAs can serve as a marker of microbial load and allow the activation status of keratinocytes to shift toward either tolerance or inflammation [48]. Keratinocytes are actively involved in the immune system and constitutively express AMPs such as cathelicidin and β-defensins 1 and 3 [37]. This expression of AMPs, as well as of cytokines and chemokines, can be quickly increased when keratinocyte pattern recognition receptors (PRRs) such as Toll-like receptor 2 (TLR2) detect bacterial lipoproteins, nucleic acids, and cell wall components [37]. This results in direct antimicrobial effects as well as recruitment and education of additional immune cells involved in innate and adaptive immunity including dendritic cells, macrophages, mast cells, natural killer cells, and a wide variety of T cells [37].

In addition to modifying keratinocyte behavior, the skin's resident microorganisms can help with wound healing and in strengthening the epidermal barrier [37, 48]. *S. epidermidis* is relatively unique in its ability to recruit and affect the function of cytotoxic T cells, using these effector T cells to modulate keratinocyte behaviors in wound healing and defense against pathogens [48]. After skin wounding, *S. epidermidis* inhibited TLR3-driven inflammatory cytokine production in cultured keratinocytes, reducing levels of inflammation [9, 33, 37]. In addition, activation of TLR2 in keratinocytes by *S. epidermidis* increases the tight junction barrier in cultured keratinocytes, helping maintaining barrier homeostasis [37]. *S. epidermidis* produces antibacterial peptides (bacteriocins) which prohibit colonization with pathogenic strains of *S. aureus* and other potential pathogens [2].

Staphylococcus epidermidis, which comprises more than 90% of all aerobic resident microbiota, does have the potential to cause serious infections, but primarily acts as a key commensal for healthy skin function. Of note, *S. epidermidis* is more than a single microbe; individual strains vary significantly in their genome content, functional potential, and relationship to the host immune system [48]. *S. epidermidis* produces peptides called phenol-soluble modulins (PSMs) that have potent antimicrobial functions that can selectively kill the skin pathogens *Streptococcus pyogenes*, *Escherichia coli*, and *S. aureus*—even inhibiting *S. aureus* biofilm formation while not harming other *S. epidermidis* [2, 6, 37]. PSMs produced by *S. epidermidis* and *Propionibacterium* species cooperate with host-derived AMPs (antimicrobial peptides made by keratinocytes, including β-defensin 2 and cathelicidin) to promote neutrophil recruitment and increase bacterial killing [8]. AMPs are abundant on skin and can reduce pathogens in even nano-molar amounts [6, 8]. PSMs can also be incorporated into neutrophil extracellular traps (NETs), which are another innate host defense against infection [6, 9, 37]. *Staphylococcus aureus* strains also produce PSMs, but these have minimal antimicrobial activity and instead induce lysis of neutrophils, whereas *S. epidermidis* PSMs have bacteria-killing activity but do not harm neutrophils [6].

Other commensal bacterial functions have also been characterized. *C. acnes* is capable of inhibiting MRSA by fermenting glycerol, a metabolite that naturally occurs in the skin, into a number of short-chain fatty acids that result in a decreased intracellular pH within *S. aureus* to inhibit its growth [37]. In addition, *Propionibacterium* species and other gram-positive bacteria increase keratinocyte expression of AMPs [6]. *C. acnes* and *Staphylococcus epidermidi*s can make antimicrobial free fatty acids by hydrolyzing sebum triglycerides and thus lower the pH of the skin surface [3]. This makes the skin inhospitable for pathogens such as *S. aureus* and *Streptococcus pyogenes* but allows less virulent coagulase-negative *Staphylococcus* and *Corynebacterium* to flourish [3].

Staphylococcus aureus is a common pathogen in skin diseases and systemic infections; however, *S. aureus* colonizes the skin of about 20–30% of the population [49]. *S. aureus* is relatively resistant to host defenses due to alterations in the charge of the bacterial cell surface, production of defensin-blocking staphylokinase, and formation of cathelicidin-cleaving aureolysin [49]. *S. aureus* is also able to evade phagocytes by inhibiting opsonization and by scavenging free radicals [49]. Unfortunately, there have emerged many antibiotic-resistant strains, including methicillin-resistant *S. aureus* (MRSA), as well as resistance to kanamycin, tobramycin, bleomycin, tetracycline, and vancomycin [49]. Use of topical probiotics may have a role in decreasing *S. aureus* burden; for example, *C. acnes* can function as a probiotic that suppresses growth of *S. aureus*, in particular community-acquired MRSA, through fermentation of glycerol [50].

Dysbiosis of the Skin Microbiome

Skin microbiota change the most rapidly, followed by gut and then oral sites [7]. The impact of environmental factors such as climate, temperature, UV exposure, lifestyle, and nutritional status on microbial communities needs further characterization [38]. Frequent hand washing has been reported to disturb the skin barrier, resulting in skin irritation and changes in the hand microbiome; cosmetics, hygiene products, makeup, and moisturizers have also been implicated in modifying the skin microbiome [38]. Antibiotics, radiotherapy, and chemotherapy may also impact microbiota [38]. Shifting of microbial communities that alter host–microbiome interactions can been associated with disease [9]. However, it is not always clear if dysbiosis leads to skin disease or if it is seen as a consequence [37].

While most cutaneous microorganisms are harmless and even beneficial, some resident microorganisms are potentially pathogenic under certain conditions and are referred to as "pathobionts" [8]. The distinction between harmless or pathogenic lies not only in the inherent properties of the microbe but in the health of the skin ecosystem, barrier integrity, and other interrelated local factors [2]. Biofilms are multicellular, surface-attached agglomerations of microorganisms whose regulation involves quorum-sensing systems. Biofilm state bacteria present different metabolic and physiological functions that render them more virulent and resistant to antibiotics [51]. Biofilm formation is an essential staphylococcal virulence factor [9]. Biofilms can also be made by *S. aureus*, *S. epidermidis*, *C. acnes*, and *Malassezia* [51].

Acne and the Skin Microbiome

Acne vulgaris (AV) is absent in non-Westernized individuals in Papua New Guinea and Paraguay and rare in some other communities with hunter–gatherer diets [4, 9]. In most Westernized countries, the incidence of acne is up to 80%, and it is speculated that the high glycemic index loads in the Western diet could lead to increased androgens, increased insulin-like growth factor-1, and altered retinoid signaling [4, 9]. AV is correlated with a surge in androgens that influence sebum production, cellular differentiation, altered keratinization, proliferation, lipogenesis, and comedogenesis in sebocytes and keratinocytes [33], as well as the host inflammatory response, thought to contribute to the inflammatory acne lesions [43].

Puberty-associated development of sebaceous glands coincides with age-related increased skin colonization with *Actinobacteria* such as *Propionibacterium* (comprising 90% of the pilosebaceous unit) and *Corynebacterium* [43, 52]. These altered follicles are then thought to be primed to develop acne lesions under certain circumstances, such as altered bacterial colonization and association with *C. acnes* [9].

C. acnes is an aerotolerant, anaerobic bacterium that is susceptible to ultraviolet radiation and is found in greatest density deep in the partially anoxic follicles [3]. *C. acnes* survives by breaking down triglycerides in sebum, releasing free fatty acids (FFAs), and obtaining energy in the process [3]. *C. acnes* also secretes porphyrins, which oxidize squalene, and this combination of FFAs and oxidized squalene acidify and weaken the skin and promote comedo formation [33, 43].

Interestingly, one study demonstrated that samples from patients with acne had higher amounts of *C. acnes* and more follicles containing *C. acnes* compared to control samples [9]. However, in another study, acne-affected skin versus healthy skin showed no difference in relative abundance of *C. acnes*, but certain *C. acnes* strains, based on their phylotype, were highly associated with acne [53]. On healthy skin, those strains were less abundant, and other strains were more prevalent [53]. These acne-associated strains carry unique genetic elements, not present in the strains associated with healthy individuals, which may contribute to virulence and pathogenicity, although the methods of this study have been questioned as to whether true deductions can be made [53,

54]. The sebum of acne patients contains a higher amount of squalene peroxide and decreased vitamin E, which may contribute to the growth of different *C. acnes* strains [33]. Two strains classified as ribotype 4 and ribotype 5 were unique only to acne patients; both carried similar genetic elements and are now thought to play a role in the pathogenesis of the disease [53]. While *C. acnes* was found to be the predominant species (87%) in healthy skin, follicles afflicted with acne are colonized by multiple other bacterial species, including other commensal microorganisms, such as *Staphylococcus epidermidis*, *Propionibacterium humerusii*, and *P. granulosum* [53, 55].

Acne-associated *C. acnes* strains induce significant inflammatory responses in keratinocytes, sebocytes, and peripheral blood mononuclear cells, and this does not occur in non-acne-associated strains [43]. Biofilm formation by *C. acnes* may contribute to keratinocyte adhesion and activation of insulin-like growth factor-1 receptor signaling and upregulation of filaggrin, causing keratinocyte differentiation and proliferation, and ultimately comedone formation [43, 51]. *C. acnes* strains associated with acne produced more porphyrins and were stronger biofilm producers, traits that may confer protection from antibiotics and promote more invasive infections [43, 51]. Vitamin B12 supplementation alters the transcriptional activities and increases porphyrin production in acne-associated *C. acnes* strains, while health-associated *C. acnes* strains do not respond to vitamin B12 supplementation [43].

C. acnes then further induces inflammation in acne via binding of TLR-2 and TLR-4 on keratinocytes and inducing subsequent inflammatory cascades such as through monocytes, activates complement, and promotes conversion of naive T cells into Th 17 cells [43]. Local epithelial injury and inflammation ensues with the secretion of hyaluronidases, lipases, phosphatases, and proteases and induction of matrix metalloproteinases [9, 43].

Several studies suggest that *C. acnes* can be inhibited by *S. epidermidis* through production of succinic acid, which has anti-*C. acnes* activity, and production of polymorphic toxins that are antibacterial [43]. Additionally, *S. epidermidis* secretes staphylococcal lipoteichoic acid, which could reduce *C. acnes*-associated inflammation by indirectly inhibiting TLR-2 expression in keratinocytes [43, 48]. Furthermore, *S. epidermidis* abundance is shown to increase at the expense of *C. acnes*, suggesting that staphylococci, especially *S. epidermidis*, may protect skin against acne, but further studies are needed to confirm this [43].

Malassezia may also induce acne, and acne lesions have been shown to be significantly reduced after administration of antifungal drugs [43]. It is speculated that *Malassezia* species might switch to a pathogenic state when its growth is not controlled, leading to impaired skin barrier function, inducing inflammation and hyperproliferation of skin cells [9]. Some have proposed that *Malassezia*, whose lipase activity is ~100 times that of *C. acnes*, is the cause of refractory acne. *Malassezia restricta* and *Malassezia globosa* can be isolated from young acne patients [43]. Further study of this potential pathobiont is warranted.

One small study by Chien et al. looked at four female acne patients undergoing therapy with oral minocycline 100 mg twice daily for 4 weeks. The study showed an initial decrease from baseline of bacterial diversity followed by varying recovery rates at 1 week and 8 weeks after stopping therapy. A 1.4-fold reduction in *C. acnes* was seen with recovery following cessation of treatment. There was a transient 5.6-fold increase in *Pseudomonas* species immediately following antibiotic treatment, as well as a persistent 1.7-fold increase in the relative abundance of *Streptococcus* species, and 4.7-fold decrease in the relative abundance of *Lactobacillus* species 8 weeks following antibiotic treatment withdrawal [56].

The presence of resistant strains of *C. acnes* to antibiotics such as erythromycin (over 50%), azithromycin (82–100%), and clindamycin (90%) can manifest as a recurrence of acne after antibiotic therapy [43]. Furthermore, when patients are treated again with antibiotics, the efficacy of such drugs can be reduced or voided. A high proportion (52%) of acne patients carry at least one *C. acnes* strain resistant to clindamycin, and when topical clindamycin was administered for 16 weeks for acne treatment, the amount of resistant *C. acnes* was increased by 16 times from the baseline [43]. The use of macrolides for acne has led to at least 30% of the *S. epidermidis* from acne patients to also show resistance to erythromycin and clindamycin [43]. Mono-therapy with topical erythromycin also led to a relative abundance of *S. aureus* of the nostrils, from 15% to 40% [43].

Doxycycline resistance is also on the rise, and to a much lesser degree, minocycline resistance has been observed [43]. Other antibiotics, including trimethoprim-sulfamethoxazole, levofloxacin, rifampin, dapsone, and metronidazole have also been used for acne [43]. Gram-negative folliculitis and pharyngitis are also associated with antibiotic therapy of acne and likely are opportunistic infections resulting from disturbed microbial community ecology on the skin and in the airways, respectively [52]. Newer tetracyclines such as lymecycline and sarecycline are now available, and how they may impact the skin microbiome is yet to be determined.

Given the above findings and increasing antibiotic resistance among *C. acnes* and *S. epidermidis* strains to macrolides (such as erythromycin, clarithromycin, azithromycin) and clindamycin (a lincosamide) worldwide, replacing antibiotics with therapies that do not place selective pressures on our commensal microbiota is critically important. In addition, to reduce the emergence of antibiotic resistance, it is currently recommended that topical antibiotics be used in combination with benzoyl peroxide (BPO) or a retinoid in acne treatment. It is also recommended that oral antibiotics not be used longer than 12 weeks. Studies have shown that combining clindamycin with BPO or retinoid for topical application not only significantly reduced the total number of *C. acnes* on the skin but also lowered antibiotic resistance of *C. acnes* to erythromycin and clindamycin [43].

Probiotic topical application with a beneficial microorganism may have a role in the treatment of acne. Topical probiotics have been shown to modify the skin barrier and increase the antimicrobial properties of the skin [57]. *Streptococcus thermophiles* has high levels of neutral sphingomyelinase, which may lead to sphingomyelin hydrolysis [58]. When the bacteria were applied as a cream for 2 weeks on elderly women's forearms, it led to a significant increase of stratum corneum ceramide levels [59]. Additionally, the ceramide phytosphingosine (PS) can exhibit direct antimicrobial activity against *C. acnes* [57]. A pilot study of the clinical application of 0.2% PS versus placebo over 60 days revealed an 89% reduction of acneiform papules and pustules [60]. Additionally, succinic acid, a fatty acid fermentation product of *Staphylococcus epidermidis*, can inhibit the growth of *C. acnes* [50]. Strain K12 of *S. salivarius* and *L. paracasei* NCC2461 have been shown to inhibit inflammatory pathways on epithelium and could also be candidates for further study in acne [57].

A randomized, double-blinded, placebo-controlled trial studied the use of a lotion containing *Enterococcus faecalis*, which makes an enterocin that is highly bacteriocidal against *C. acnes*, over 8 weeks in patients with mild to moderate acne [61]. The study showed a statistically significant reduction of inflammatory pustular lesions, but not of comedones, compared to placebo [61]. A reduction in acne count, size, and associated erythema and improved skin barrier repair and reduced ski microflora was again noted during a clinical study of *Lactobacillus plantarum* 5% extract, but not at 1% [57].

Another potential therapeutic could involve topical prebiotics, such as glucomannans, which have been found to stimulate the immune system and the growth of beneficial probiotic microorganisms, such as *Lactobacillus*, while inhibiting undesirable bacteria [62]. An in vitro study showed that the growth of *Propionibacterium acnes* was inhibited by various *Lactobacillus* strains in probiotics, and this inhibition was enhanced significantly in the presence of konjac glucomannan hydrolysates [62].

Correcting microbiome dysbiosis by application of commensal skin bacteria is an area for further research. In addition, vaccines for acne using bacterial targets are also being explored [43]. Given the degree of diversity in an individual's cutaneous microbiome, topical prebiotics, probiotics, and vaccines will most likely be adjuvants in a broader therapeutic plan that will include changes in lifestyle, diet, hygiene practices, and more [63].

Recommendations of Oral Acne Treatments

- Increased fiber (greater than 20 g a day)
- Probiotics
  - *Lactobacillus rhamnosus* SP1
  - *Lactobacillus acidophilus*, *Lactobacillus delbrueckii* subspecies *bulgaricus*, and *Bifidobacterium bifidum*
- Green tea extract
- Gugulipid
- Sunder Vati
- Some Ayurvedic plant extracts

Rosacea and Skin Microbiome

Rosacea can be divided into four subtypes: erythematotelangiectatic, papulopustular, phymatous, and ocular; these subtypes are based on specific clinical manifestations and morphologic characteristics [64]. Abnormal sebaceous glands, changes in the cutaneous vascular and lymphatic system, and dermal matrix degeneration are thought to all play a role in the pathophysiology of rosacea [64].

In addition to *Malassezia* and *Propionibacterium*, the sebaceous unit is colonized by *Demodex* skin mites, particularly *D. folliculorum* and *D. brevis*. This predilection may in part be explained by lipases produced by *Demodex*, allowing the mite to utilize sebum as a food source. Other nutritional sources may be cellular debris or bacteria such as *C. acnes* that reside in the pilosebaceous unit [52]. *Demodex* increases in prevalence with age, and increased density is associated with erythematotelangiectatic and papulopustular rosacea.

Demodex mites are found in increased numbers on the skin of rosacea patients; in one study, *D. folliculorum* density was 5.7 times higher in rosacea patients than in healthy volunteers [65]. In another study, *D. folliculorum* was detected at a tenfold increased density and in increased frequency (90% vs 12%) of the 92 rosacea subjects [66]. Accordingly, a higher gene expression rate for pro-inflammatory cytokines and broad immune system activation was noted with increased numbers of mites [65]. An inverse relationship between *D. folliculorum* density and inflammation markers in the skin of rosacea patients has also been observed, with differences observed between rosacea subtypes [65]. Hair follicle infestation was associated with intense perifollicular infiltrate of predominantly (90–95%) CD4 helper/inducer T cells [66]. Increased number of macrophages and Langerhans cells were only seen in those subjects with a positive *D. folliculorum* finding [66].

Rosacea patients have abnormal activation of the innate immune pattern recognition receptors, expressing higher amounts of TLR2 than healthy subjects [9, 64]. Those with rosacea also have higher epidermal expression of TLR2 than healthy subjects, triggering a pattern of abnormal production of cathelicidin antimicrobial peptides and increased expression and activity of serine protease kallikrein that is characteristic in rosacea [9,64]. Additionally, the *Demodex*-associated microbiota, in particular *Bacillus oleronius*, which is not typically found in the commensal skin microbiota, triggers rosacea-like inflammation [52].

While *Demodex* mites do not seem to be the sole cause of rosacea, they may represent an important cofactor, especially in papulopustular rosacea [66]. Immunohistochemical findings suggest that a delayed hypersensitivity reaction, possibly triggered by antigens of follicular origin, probably related to *D. folliculorum*, may occur, stimulating progression of the affection to the papulopustular stage [66]. Mites may play a role in exacerbation of rosacea either by disrupting the skin barrier or by triggering TLR2 activation through chitin in the insect cuticle or by the bacteria that live in the digestive tract of *Demodex* that is released into surrounding tissues, triggering further tissue degradation and inflammation [9]. A genetic predisposition in the host changes ecological characteristics in the skin, influencing a shift in the microbiome, and *Demodex* may take advantage of these changes, evoking a response which makes the skin susceptible to UV exposure, alcohol, hormone fluctuations, and bacterial overgrowth (such as *S epidermidis*) on developing papules [9]. Age-specific modulations of TLR expression might play an essential role in the course rosacea as well [9].

Because *Demodex* are present on healthy skin, and considered as part of the commensal microbiota, it is likely that host status contributes to their transition from commensal to potential pathogen. However, additional research is needed to provide insight into the mechanism in which microorganisms, including *Demodex*, influence the pathogenesis of rosacea [52].

Future Directions

The interrelatedness of the microbiome with the gastrointestinal tract, brain, and skin functions has been termed the gut–brain–skin axis, and studies are showing that many metabolic, immune, neurological, and endocrine processes appear to be regulated by gut and skin microbiota [67]. The gut–brain–skin axis hypothesis led to investigations of oral pre- and probiotics for the skin, and a new generation of emollients and moisturizers has now been developed, including lysates of bacteria, such as *Vitreoscilla filiformis* or *Lactobacillus* [38]. It is possible that one day microbes will be used to restore certain functions to the gut or skin that are deficient or abnormal in the host [68]. Success of fecal microbiota transplantation for the treatment of *C. difficile* colitis highlights the therapeutic potential of microbial manipulation. The role of probiotics, prebiotics, bacteriotherapy, and use of bacteriophages in the skin for rosacea and acne is yet to be determined [12].

The association of the human microbiome with the macrobiome of our environment provides a link between our physiology and how it is affected by our surroundings. The holobiont perspective is one in which humans are a multispecies entity and provides key insights for practicing truly integrative medicine, where environment, diet, and biology are all factors in optimizing global health [2]. Loss of biodiversity through environmental degradation and loss of contact with "green space," whether by climate change, invasive species, or industrial activity, is linked to many disease states and poorer mental health [2]. Thus, while individual therapy for given diseases such as acne or rosacea will continue to play a role, a broader view of our interaction with nature and the environment may become even more critical to help heal microbiome-associated conditions.

References

1. Lloyd-Price J, Abu-Ali G, Huttenhower C. The healthy human microbiome. Genome Med. 2016;8:51.
2. Prescott SL, Larcombe DL, Logan AC, West C, Burks W, Caraballo L, et al. The skin microbiome: impact of modern environments on skin ecology, barrier integrity, and systemic immune programming. World Allergy Organ J. 2017;10:29.
3. Ladizinski B, McLean R, Lee KC, Elpern DJ, Eron L. The human skin microbiome. Int J Dermatol. 2014;53:1177–9.
4. Weyrich LS, Dixit S, Farrer AG, Cooper AJ, Cooper AJ. The skin microbiome: associations between altered microbial communities and disease. Australas J Dermatol. 2015;56:268–74.
5. Zeeuwen PLJM, Kleerebezem M, Timmerman HM, Schalkwijk J. Microbiome and skin diseases. Curr Opin Allergy Clin Immunol. 2013;13:514–20.
6. Chen YE, Tsao H. The skin microbiome: current perspectives and future challenges. J Am Acad Dermatol. 2013;69:143–55.
7. Gilbert JA, Blaser MJ, Caporaso JG, Jansson JK, Lynch SV, Knight R. Current understanding of the human microbiome. Nat Med. 2018;24:392–400.
8. Yamazaki Y, Nakamura Y, Núñez G. Role of the microbiota in skin immunity and atopic dermatitis. Allergol Int. 2017;66:539–44.

9. Schommer NN, Gallo RL. Structure and function of the human skin microbiome. Trends Microbiol. 2013;21:660–8.
10. Pflughoeft KJ, Versalovic J. Human microbiome in health and disease. Annu Rev Pathol. 2012;7:99–122.
11. Muszer M, Noszczyńska M, Kasperkiewicz K, Skurnik M. Human microbiome: when a friend becomes an enemy. Arch Immunol Ther Exp. 2015;63:287–98.
12. Kong HH, Segre JA. The molecular revolution in cutaneous biology: investigating the skin microbiome. J Invest Dermatol. 2017;137:e119–22.
13. Baba H, Masuyama A, Yoshimura C, Aoyama Y, Takano T, Ohki K. Oral intake of lactobacillus helveticus-fermented milk whey decreased transepidermal water loss and prevented the onset of sodium dodecylsulfate-induced dermatitis in mice. Biosci Biotechnol Biochem. 2010;74:18–23.
14. Philippe D, Blum S, Benyacoub J. Oral Lactobacillus paracasei improves skin barrier function recovery and reduces local skin inflammation. Eur J Dermatol. 2011;21:279–80.
15. Gueniche A, Philippe D, Bastien P, Reuteler G, Blum S, Castiel-Higounenc I, et al. Randomised double-blind placebo-controlled study of the effect of Lactobacillus paracasei NCC 2461 on skin reactivity. Benef Microbes. 2014;5:137–45.
16. Benyacoub J, Bosco N, Blanchard C, Demont A, Philippe D, Castiel-Higounenc I, et al. Immune modulation property of Lactobacillus paracasei NCC2461 (ST11) strain and impact on skin defences. Benef Microbes. 2014;5:129–36.
17. Poutahidis T, Kearney SM, Levkovich T, Qi P, Varian BJ, Lakritz JR, et al. Microbial symbionts accelerate wound healing via the neuropeptide hormone oxytocin. PLoS One. 2013;e78898:8.
18. Salem I, Ramser A, Isham N, Ghannoum MA. The gut microbiome as a major regulator of the gut-skin axis. Front Microbiol. 2018;9:1459.
19. Fabbrocini G, Bertona M, Picazo Ó, Pareja-Galeano H, Monfrecola G, Emanuele E. Supplementation with Lactobacillus rhamnosus SP1 normalises skin expression of genes implicated in insulin signalling and improves adult acne. Benef Microbes. 2016;7:625–30.
20. Bowe W, Patel NB, Logan AC. Acne vulgaris, probiotics and the gut-brain-skin axis: from anecdote to translational medicine. Benef Microbes. 2014;5:185–99.
21. Stokes JH, Pillsbury DM. The effect on the skin of emotional and nervous states: III. Theoretical and practical consideration

of a gastro-intestinal mechanism. Arch Dermatol Syphilol. 1930;22:962–93.

22. Deng Y, Wang H, Zhou J, Mou Y, Wang G, Xiong X. Patients with acne vulgaris have a distinct gut microbiota in comparison with healthy controls. Acta Derm Venereol. 2018;98:783–90.
23. Yan H-M, Zhao H-J, Guo D-Y, Zhu P-Q, Zhang C-L, Jiang W. Gut microbiota alterations in moderate to severe acne vulgaris patients. J Dermatol. 2018;45:1166–71.
24. Marchetti F, Capizzi R, Tulli A. Efficacy of regulators of the intestinal bacterial flora in the therapy of acne vulgaris. Clin Ter. 1987;122:339–43. [In Italian].
25. Volkova LA, Khalif IL, Kabanova IN. Impact of the impaired intestinal microflora on the course of acne vulgaris. Klin Med. 2001;79:39–41.
26. Jung GW, Tse JE, Guiha I, Rao J. Prospective, randomized, open-label trial comparing the safety, efficacy, and tolerability of an acne treatment regimen with and without a probiotic supplement and minocycline in subjects with mild to moderate acne. J Cutan Med Surg. 2013;7:114–22.
27. Clark AK, Haas KN, Sivamani RK. Edible plants and their influence on the gut microbiome and acne. Int J Mol Sci. 2017;18(5):E1070. https://doi.org/10.3390/ijms18051070.
28. Lu PH, Hsu CH. Does supplementation with green tea extract improve acne in post-adolescent women? A randomized, double-blind, and placebo-controlled clinical trial. Complement Ther Med. 2016;25:159–63.
29. Thappa DM, Dogra J. (1994) Nodulocystic acne: oral gugulipid versus tetracycline. J Dermatol. 1994;21:729–31.
30. He J-M, Mu Q. The medicinal uses of the genus Mahonia in traditional Chinese medicine: an ethnopharmacological, phytochemical and pharmacological review. J Ethnopharmacol. 2015;175:668–83.
31. Egeberg A, Weinstock LB, Thyssen EP, Gislason GH, Thyssen JP. Rosacea and gastrointestinal disorders: a population-based cohort study. Br J Dermatol. 2017;176:100–6.
32. Drago F, De Col E, Agnoletti AF, Schiavetti I, Savarino V, Rebora A, et al. The role of small intestinal bacterial overgrowth in rosacea: a 3-year follow-up. J Am Acad Dermatol. 2016;75:e113–5.
33. Musthaq S, Mazuy A, Jakus J. The microbiome in dermatology. Clin Dermatol. 2018;36:390–8.
34. Kendall SN. Remission of rosacea induced by reduction of gut transit time. Clin Exp Dermatol. 2004;29:297–9.

35. Nam J-H, Yun Y, Kim H-S, Kim H-N, Jung HJ, Chang Y, et al. Rosacea and its association with enteral microbiota in Korean females. Exp Dermatol. 2018;27:37–42.
36. Fortuna MC, Garelli V, Pranteda G, Romaniello F, Cardone M, Carlesimo M, et al. A case of scalp rosacea treated with low dose doxycycline and probiotic therapy and literature review on therapeutic options. Dermatol Ther. 2016;29:249–51.
37. Sanford JA, Gallo RL. Functions of the skin microbiota in health and disease. Semin Immunol. 2013;25:370–7.
38. Dréno B, Araviiskaia E, Berardesca E, Gontijo G, Sanchez Viera M, Xiang LF, et al. Microbiome in healthy skin, update for dermatologists. J Eur Acad Dermatol Venereol. 2016;30:2038–47.
39. Capone K. Intra and interpersonal changes in the skin microbiome from infancy to adulthood. Presented at 2013 AAP National Conference and Exhibition. Available at: https://aap.confex.com/aap/2013/webprogram/Paper21199.html.
40. Grice EA, Segre JA. The skin microbiome. Nat Rev Microbiol. 2011;9:244–53.
41. Schloss PD. An integrated view of the skin microbiome. Nature. 2014;514:44–5.
42. Grice EA, Kong HH, Conlan S, Deming CB, Davis J, Young AC, et al. Topographical and temporal diversity of the human skin microbiome. Science. 2009;324:1190–2.
43. Xu H, Li H. Acne, the skin microbiome, and antibiotic treatment. Am J Clin Dermatol. 2019;20(3):335–44. https://doi.org/10.1007/s40257-018-00417-3.
44. Cosseau C, Romano-Bertrand S, Duplan H, Lucas O, Ingrassia I, Pigasse C, et al. Proteobacteria from the human skin microbiota: species-level diversity and hypotheses. One Health. 2016;2:33–41.
45. Grice EA, Kong HH, Renaud G, Young AC, Bouffard GG, Blakesley RW, et al. A diversity profile of the human skin microbiota. Genome Res. 2008;18:1043–50.
46. Hannigan GD, Meisel JS, Tyldsley AS, Zheng Q, Hodkinson BP, SanMiguel AJ, et al. The human skin double-stranded DNA virome: topographical and temporal diversity, genetic enrichment, and dynamic associations with the host microbiome. MBio. 2015;6:e01578–15.
47. Hall JB, Cong Z, Imamura-Kawasawa Y, Kidd BA, Dudley JT, Thiboutot DM, et al. Isolation and identification of the follicular microbiome: implications for acne research. J Invest Dermatol. 2018;138:2033–40.

48. Stacy A, Belkaid Y. Microbial guardians of skin health. Science. 2019;363:227–8.
49. Cogen AL, Nizet V, Gallo RL. Skin microbiota: a source of disease or defence? Br J Dermatol. 2008;158:442–55.
50. Shu M, Wang Y, Yu J, Kuo S, Coda A, Jiang Y, Gallo RL, Huang CM. Fermentation of Propionibacterium acnes, a commensal bacterium in the human skin microbiome, as skin probiotics against methicillin-resistant Staphylococcus aureus. PLoS One. 2013;8:e55380.
51. Brandwein M, Steinberg D, Meshner S. Microbial biofilms and the human skin microbiome. NPJ Biofilms Microbiomes. 2016;2:3.
52. Grice EA. The skin microbiome: potential for novel diagnostic and therapeutic approaches to cutaneous disease. Semin Cutan Med Surg. 2014;33:98–103.
53. Fitz-Gibbon S, Tomida S, Chiu BH, Nguyen L, Du C, Liu M, et al. Propionibacterium acnes strain populations in the human skin microbiome associated with acne. J Invest Dermatol. 2013;133:2152–60.
54. Eady EA, Layton AM. A distinct acne microbiome: fact or fiction? J Invest Dermatol. 2013;133:2294–5.
55. Bek-Thomsen M, Lomholt HB, Kilian M. Acne is not associated with yet-uncultured bacteria. J Clin Microbiol. 2008;46:3355–60.
56. Chien AL, Tsai J, Leung S, Mongodin EF, Nelson AM, Kang S, et al. Association of systemic antibiotic treatment of acne with skin microbiota characteristics. JAMA Dermatol. 2019;155(4):425–34. https://doi.org/10.1001/jamadermatol.2018.5221.
57. Kober MM, Bowe WP. The effect of probiotics on immune regulation, acne, and photoaging. Int J Womens Dermatol. 2015;1:85–9.
58. Marzio LD, Di Marzio L, Cinque B, De Simone C, Grazia CM. Effect of the lactic acid bacterium streptococcus thermophilus on ceramide levels in human keratinocytes in vitro and stratum corneum in vivo. J Invest Dermatol. 1999;113:98–106.
59. Dimarzio L, Cinque B, Cupelli F, De Simone C, Cifone MG. Giuliani MIncrease of skin-ceramide levels in aged subjects following a short-term topical application of bacterial sphingomyelinase from streptococcus thermophilus. Int J Immunopathol Pharmacol. 2008;21:137–43.
60. Pavicic T, Wollenweber U, Farwick M, Korting HC. Antimicrobial and -inflammatory activity and efficacy of phytosphin-

gosine: an in vitro and in vivo study addressing acne vulgaris. Int J Cosmet Sci. 2007;29:181–90.
61. Kang BS, Seo JG, Lee GS, Kim JH, Kim SY, Han YW, et al. Antimicrobial activity of Enterocins from enterococcus faecalis SL-5 against Propionibacterium acnes, the causative agent in acne vulgaris, and its therapeutic effect. J Microbiol. 2009;47:101–9.
62. Al-Ghazzewi FH, Tester RF. Effect of konjac glucomannan hydrolysates and probiotics on the growth of the skin bacterium Propionibacterium acnes in vitro. Int J Cosmet Sci. 2010;32:139–42.
63. Tavaria F. Topical use of probiotics: the natural balance. Porto Biomed J. 2017;2:69–70.
64. Picardo M, Ottaviani M. Skin microbiome and skin disease: the example of rosacea. J Clin Gastroenterol. 2014;48(Suppl 1):S85–6.
65. Casas C, Paul C, Lahfa M, Livideanu B, Lejeune O, Alvarez-Georges S, et al. Quantification of Demodex folliculorum by PCR in rosacea and its relationship to skin innate immune activation. Exp Dermatol. 2012;21:906–10.
66. Georgala S, Katoulis AC, Kylafis GD, Koumantaki-Mathioudaki E, Georgala C, Aroni K. Increased density of Demodex folliculorum and evidence of delayed hypersensitivity reaction in subjects with papulopustular rosacea. J Eur Acad Dermatol Venereol. 2001;15:441–4.
67. Arck P, Handjiski B, Hagen E, Pincus M, Bruenahl C, Bienenstock J, et al. Is there a "gut-brain-skin axis"? Exp Dermatol. 2010;19:401–5.
68. Dorrestein PC, Gallo RL, Knight R. Microbial skin inhabitants: friends forever. Cell. 2016;165:771–2.

Chapter 2
Vitamins and Minerals in the Treatment of Acne Vulgaris

Justin W. Marson and Hilary E. Baldwin

Introduction

Numerous pathogenic factors are thought to be important in acne, providing many targets for therapeutic intervention. The presence of *Cutibacterium acnes*, follicular hyperkeratinization, altered sebum production, the production of pro-inflammatory cytokines, and the resulting inflammatory response are well documented. Sebum production, under the influence of androgens, is abnormal in terms of both quantity and quality, and the sebaceous glands also produce antimicrobial peptides and inflammatory cytokines. Lipoteichoic acid from the wall of *C. acnes* binds to toll-like receptor 2 which induces pro-inflammatory cytokines via activation of nuclear factor kappa B (NF-kB). Steps along each of these pathways provide a multitude of opportunities for vitamins and minerals to interact and disrupt the inflammatory march of acne.

J. W. Marson
Internal Medicine, University of California, Irvine Medical Center, Orange, CA, USA

H. E. Baldwin (✉)
Department of Dermatology, Rutgers Robert Wood Johnson, Piscataway, NJ, USA
e-mail: hbaldwin@acnetrc.com

R. N. Rupani, P. A. Lio (eds.), *Integrative Dermatology*,
https://doi.org/10.1007/978-3-030-58954-7_2

Vitamins

A vitamin is an essential micronutrient (or group of molecules) that is required for the functioning of an organism. Vitamins cannot be synthesized by the organism and must be obtained from sources outside the body. These varied sources may include food, fortified foods, supplements, and, in the cases of vitamin D and K, sunshine and the gut flora, respectively. Vitamins also have diverse functions. Vitamin A regulates both cell differentiation and growth. The B complex vitamins act as enzyme cofactors or precursors for energy metabolism. Vitamins C and E function primarily as antioxidants, while vitamin D serves as a prohormone that regulates mineral metabolism.

We must remember that while vitamin supplementation is often beneficial, hypervitaminosis is possible, with the fat-soluble vitamins A, D, E, and K leading to toxicity from accumulation. The water-soluble vitamins B and C are readily excreted in the urine; therefore, vitamin B and C toxicity is unlikely, and consistent intake is important.

Vitamin A

Vitamin A is not a single entity, but rather a group of fat-soluble retinoids (e.g., retinal, retinol, and retinyl esters) that support and regulate both cell differentiation and cell growth. Within the body, retinyl palmitate is converted into retinol, which in turn is converted into retinaldehyde and finally retinoic acid. Active ingredients that are more biochemically similar to retinoic acid are more readily converted to retinoic acid and are, therefore, more efficacious. Beta carotene and other carotenoids are provitamins that must be metabolized into vitamin A.

The skin is one of the major retinoid-responsive tissues in the body, as cells in both the epidermis and dermis contain retinoid receptors. Long-term use of topical retinoids has well-known applications for skin health, including antiaging, scar improvement, improving dyspigmentation, and the treatment of acne. Of note, only retinoic acid has been shown to benefit acne.

Topical retinoids help to normalize the hyperkeratinization (i.e., altered growth and differentiation of follicular keratinocytes) implicated in acne pathophysiology by reducing keratinocyte proliferation, promoting keratinocyte differentiation, and increasing follicular epithelial turnover [1, 2]. Retinoids also inhibit inflammation by suppressing toll-like receptors, leukocyte migration, and the AP-1 pathway [3].

Oral supplementation with vitamin A is not effective for acne in sub-toxic doses. Excessive intake of preformed vitamin A has been linked to hepatotoxicity and teratogenicity in both human and animals [4]. As carotenoids are provitamins, they are less likely to cause toxicity. The daily recommended dose of preformed vitamin A is 2700 IU for women, while doses exceeding 10,000 IU have been linked to teratogenicity in human and animals [5].

Vitamin D

Vitamin D is a fat-soluble vitamin naturally present in very few foods. As a result, it is often added to “fortify” foods or taken as a dietary supplement. Exposure to ultraviolet light also triggers vitamin D synthesis in the skin. Dermally derived and dietary vitamin D is then further biochemically activated by the liver and kidneys. Vitamin D acts as a prohormone steroid in the body and plays numerous roles within endocrine, paracrine, and autocrine functions [6]. It plays a major role in serum calcium homeostasis and modulates cell proliferation, differentiation, and apoptosis in a paracrine and autocrine manner [7]. Vitamin D also plays a role in innate and adaptive immune functions and may serve as an immune modulator in numerous dermatologic diseases such as atopic dermatitis and psoriasis and autoimmune conditions such as lupus erythematosus, inflammatory bowel disease, vitiligo, and alopecia [8–13].

Like other fat-soluble vitamins, there is an upper limit to safety. Daily ingestion of 10,000–40,000 IU/day is considered toxic, as it interferes with calcium homeostasis.

Rationale for Use in the Treatment of Acne

Vitamin D receptors are present in human sebocytes, where they may modulate lipid production [14]. In vitro studies using human sebaceous cells incubated with the active form of vitamin D (calcitriol) demonstrated a dose-dependent suppression of cell proliferation. Inhibition of sebocyte proliferation and differentiation has been shown to be a key factor in the production of sebum [15]. Vitamin D also induces TLR2, which initiates innate immune responses in the skin, resulting in antibacterial activity [16].

Vitamin D has also been shown to inhibit Th 17-mediated inflammation, a pathway that is potently exacerbated by *C. acnes* [14]. The expression of inflammatory biomarkers in cultured sebocytes has also been shown to be affected by vitamin D [17]. Together these findings suggest that vitamin D analogs may be useful in the treatment of acne via anti-inflammatory effects and suppression/alteration of sebum production.

Clinical Evidence of Vitamin D Efficacy in Acne

A correlation between liver-activated serum 25-hydroxyvitamin D (calcidiol) levels and acne has been evaluated globally in several studies, with conflicting results. At least three controlled cohort and retrospective review studies have found an inverse association between serum vitamin D levels and acne severity [18–20]. Furthermore, in one study of 80 acne and 80 healthy individuals, Lim et al. also found a negative association with inflammatory lesions [18]. However, several studies also failed to replicate these results, including a large cross-sectional study that included 714 adolescents and accounted for possible confounding variables (e.g., vitamin D supplementation within past 6 months, diet, BMI, and exercise) [21, 22].

Clinically, serum levels of vitamin D3 were shown to increase when 90 acne patients (vs. 60 controls) were treated with isotretinoin. After evaluating serum calcidiol levels, Lim et al. went on to supplement 39 deficient acne patients and noted an improvement in inflammatory lesions [18]. Jarosz and El-Sohemy were unable to show an improvement in acne in a study of 998 college women with premenstrual syndrome supplemented with vitamin D3 [23]. Physical complaints and emotional symptoms did show signs of improvement, however.

Vitamin C

What we refer to as vitamin C is actually a group of molecules composed of L-ascorbic acid, calcium ascorbate, magnesium ascorbyl phosphate, sodium ascorbate, and sodium ascorbyl phosphate [24]. Vitamin C is a water-soluble vitamin abundantly present in fruits and vegetables and is depleted when exposed to ozone and ultraviolet light. It is present in a gradient within the skin such that the epidermis has levels 425% higher than the dermis. Its primary role in the epidermis is as an antioxidant, particularly when combined with vitamin E. It also promotes collagen formation, inhibits melanogenesis, and plays a role in the differentiation of keratinocytes [25]. It has been shown to have anti-inflammatory properties in atopic dermatitis and psoriasis [26]. Topical and oral vitamin C has been evaluated for the treatment of photodamage, hyperpigmentation, barrier dysfunction, and inflammation.

Rationale for Use in the Treatment of Acne

The use of magnesium ascorbyl phosphate, a vitamin C precursor, has been shown to decrease the expression of pro-inflammatory cytokines, matrix metalloproteinases, antimicrobial peptides, toll-like receptor 4, and lipid peroxidation in cultured sebocytes [24]. This suggests that there may be a role for vitamin C in reducing inflammation in acne.

Topical vitamin C may also improve barrier dysfunction. There is increasing evidence that there is a primary barrier dysfunction in acne-prone skin. Although not generally considered a barrier-deficient condition, it has been shown that, at baseline, there is an increase in trans-epidermal water loss, a decrease in ceramide levels, and an altered microbiome [27, 28]. All of these findings are more profound as acne severity increases. In addition to the inherent barrier defect, the use of topical acne products and isotretinoin are independently associated with increased skin drying, barrier deficit, and dysbiosis [29–31]. Of note, other inflammatory dermatoses, such as atopic dermatitis and psoriasis, also have well-documented deficiencies in ceramides, the main lipids of the stratum corneum [32].

The use of topical vitamin C has been shown to enhance the production of barrier lipids, and, in one study, plasma vitamin C and total ceramide levels in the epidermis of patients with atopic dermatitis were shown to have an inverse relationship [32].

Clinical Evidence of Efficacy in Acne

Clinically, there is no data demonstrating efficacy of vitamin C in the direct treatment of acne. However, data exists regarding an inherent barrier deficit and dysbiosis in acne and additional medication-induced dryness. Numerous studies support the use of vitamin C to repair a ceramide-deficient epidermis. A combination of ascorbyl palmitate and sodium ascorbyl phosphate was shown to control facial sebum secretion in healthy female volunteers [33]. Combined with the in vitro data showing the ability of vitamin C to reduce the production of pro-inflammatory cytokines, this suggests that vitamin C may be a useful adjunctive therapy for acne.

The question remains, should vitamin C be administered topically or orally? Skin levels of vitamin C do not increase once plasma saturation is reached; therefore, additional oral dosing is not expected to improve skin levels in people who have adequate levels of vitamin C [25]. However, topical applications are a challenge, as vitamin C is not very durable, being both water-soluble easily oxidized [34]. A quality product made under strict control is therefore essential for clinical efficacy.

Vitamin E

Vitamin E is a fat-soluble group of eight compounds comprised of tocopherols and tocotrienols. It is widely available in oils and nuts, and deficiency is uncommon. In the body it functions as an antioxidant. While upward of 1000 mg/day is considered safe, doses as low as 300 mg/day can interact with aspirin, warfarin, tamoxifen, and cyclosporine A. Topically, it has a low incidence of sensitivity [35].

Clinical Evidence of Efficacy in Acne

There is no clinical data to suggest that vitamin E is specifically helpful in the treatment of acne. However, Ozuguz et al. evaluated serum levels of vitamins A, E, and zinc in 94 subjects with acne and compared this with 56 controls [36]. They found that all three were lower in the acne patients compared with controls ($P < 0.001$). They showed a negative correlation between acne severity and vitamin E and zinc levels. There is some evidence that vitamin E may help to mitigate the side effect potential of benzoyl peroxide (BP). Benzoyl peroxide use results in the formation of oxygen free radicals which, along with the depletion of antioxidants, are responsible for the side effects of the drug. When incubated with benzoyl peroxide, keratinocyte vitamin E has been shown to be depleted by 50% in the first 30 minutes [37]. In one study, BP-induced lipid peroxidation was counteracted by the addition of vitamin E [38]. Taken together, these data suggest that topical vitamin E may help to reduce the side effects of BP and replenish BP-related depletion of vitamin E in the epidermis.

Vitamin B3 (Niacin or Nicotinic Acid)

Vitamin B3 is a water-soluble essential nutrient with potent antioxidant and anti-inflammatory properties. It is found in a variety of foods, in both natural and enriched products. Nicotinamide (aka niacinamide) is the amide form of niacin and has identical vitamin function without the vasodilatory effects. Nicotinamide is a precursor for nicotinamide adenine dinucleotide (NAD), which is a coenzyme for critical oxidation–reduction reactions in the human body. Long-term safety of vitamin B3 (i.e., 3 g daily for 5 years) has been demonstrated [39]. Vitamin B3 has been shown to be useful in several dermatologic conditions, including photo- and chronological aging, psoriasis, bullous pemphigoid, melasma, and, most recently, skin cancer chemoprevention [40–44].

Rationale for Use in the Treatment of Acne

Nicotinamide has been shown to have anti-inflammatory effects due to its ability to inhibit the in vitro secretion of interleukin-8, lysosomal enzyme release, and mast cell degranulation [45, 46]. Topically, it has been shown to reduce sebum excretion rates [47]. Lastly, it has been shown to be helpful in creating and maintaining the healthy barrier function of the skin, the healthy microbiome, and may have bacteriostatic effects on *C. acnes* [46, 48].

Clinical Evidence of Vitamin B3 Efficacy in Acne

Wolacko et al. have summarized the relevant literature regarding nicotinamide use in acne [49]. They found ten studies utilizing nicotinamide either topically (8) or orally (2), as a single agent (4) or as part of a combination product or co-application (6).

Topical Use

While there are no placebo-controlled topical trials, several studies have compared nicotinamide 4% to clindamycin and found similar efficacy [50–52]. One open-label study showed improvement from baseline [50]. Four studies utilized nicotinamide 4% in combination with other ingredients including clindamycin and retinol [53–57]. In all four studies, although efficacy was noted, it is unclear which ingredient was responsible for the clinical improvement.

Oral Use

Two open-label clinical trials have utilized nicotinamide in combination for the treatment of acne [58, 59]. In combination with zinc, copper, and folic acid, nicotinamide 750 mg QD was shown to result in high patient satisfaction ratings in 198 patients with acne and rosacea (79% reported moderate to much better at 4 weeks). Subsequent addition of an unreported oral antibiotic did not improve the perceived efficacy [58]. Shalita et al. treated 235 inflammatory acne patients with a proprietary combination of nicotinamide, azelaic acid, zinc, pyridoxine, calcium, and folic acid for 8 weeks in addition to their existing acne regimen [59]. They noted a significant improvement over previous treatment at 4 and 8 weeks ($p < 0.0001$) with an 88% reduction in visible redness in inflammatory lesions and an 81% patient satisfaction rating (much/moderately better).

Safety

None of the topical or oral studies reported major adverse effects. Slight itching and burning were noted in some studies, but the incidence was not different from the control groups. Theoretically, at doses in excess of 3 g a day, nicotinamide can cause nausea, heartburn, flushing, and an elevations in transaminases [39].

Due to small sample size, lack of placebo or topical controls, and the confounding factor of combination use, it is difficult to adequately assess the true efficacy of nicotinamide in acne. Additional well-controlled studies will be necessary to confirm the favorable results seen in these preliminary reports. In the meantime, however, nicotinamide is an inexpensive agent which can be safely utilized as part of an acne regimen. Most notably, it lacks the side effect profile of existing topical and oral acne therapies and does not carry the concern regarding antibiotic resistance.

Vitamin B12

Unlike other vitamins, there is clinical evidence that vitamin B12 supplementation is associated with acne or acneiform eruptions, from case reports dating as far back as 1958 [60–65]. Serum levels of vitamin B12 have been reported to be increased in acne patients and to normalize after successful treatment [66, 67]. Recently, Kang et al. hypothesized that the association may be due to metabolic interactions involving *C. acnes* [68]. They demonstrated an increase in the production of porphyrins in *C. acnes* from cultures of the skin microbiome obtained from ten healthy individuals who were administered supplemental B12. Porphyrins are known to induce inflammation by stimulating the production of pro-inflammatory mediators [69–71]. While more evidence is necessary to prove this hypothesis, it appears reasonable to recommend that patients obtain vitamin B12 from food sources as opposed to receiving alternative forms of vitamin B12 supplementation. Admittedly, this is more difficult for vegans, as vitamin B12 is primarily derived from animal flesh and dairy products. Fortified cereal and soy products may serve as reasonable alternatives for those with dietary restrictions.

Minerals and Acne

Minerals are generally defined as naturally occurring, solid, inorganic substances. Dietary minerals can be loosely divided into two groups: macrominerals and trace minerals, which are required in large and small amounts, respectively. Macrominerals include calcium, magnesium, phosphorous, sodium, chloride, sulfur, and potassium; and important trace minerals include iron, zinc, selenium, iodine, copper, chromium, molybdenum, fluoride, and manganese. Since minerals leach into virtually everything that we eat or drink, deficiencies are uncommon, and supplementation is rarely necessary. Supplementation must be carefully considered, as there is a delicate interplay among mineral concentrations. Too much zinc, for example, can cause copper deficiency, and calcium and phosphorous need to be in careful balance for bone health.

Data, with the notable exception of zinc, are extremely scarce for the use of mineral supplementation in the treatment of acne. In most cases data are limited to a sound scientific rationale and occasional pilot study. In addition to zinc, sulfur, chromium, selenium, and clay minerals have a paucity of data to support their use.

Zinc

Zinc is an essential micronutrient that is a cofactor in more than 300 metalloenzymes and 2000 transcription factors [72]. As such, it plays a role in many aspects of health, including immune function, wound healing, protein and DNA synthesis, and cell division [73–76]. There is no zinc storage system in the body, and daily intake is necessary to maintain health. It is present in a wide variety of foods including nuts, beans, red meat, poultry, and seafood, as well as fortified breakfast and dairy products. Deficiencies are therefore uncommon in healthy individuals. The tolerable upper limit for elemental zinc is 40 mg daily when used chronically. Zinc supplements are available in gluconate, sulfate, picolinate, acetate, and citrate formulations, and each has a different percentage of elemental zinc. Gluconate and sulfate are the most readily available, and a 10 mg elemental zinc dose would require 38.5 mg and 22 mg, respectively. At the time of this writing, 30 mg daily of elemental zinc is the most widely studied dose in the literature.

Zinc supplementation must consider potential drug interactions. Iron supplementation decreases zinc levels in humans [76]. Zinc supplementation can result in copper deficiency and resultant sideroblastic anemia [77, 78]. Co-administration of quinolone or tetracycline antibiotics with zinc can result in decreased absorption of both agents [79, 80]. It is recommended that there be a 2-hour lapse between ingestion. Penicillamine absorption is decreased by co-administration with zinc as well [80]. Lastly, hydrochlorothiazide treatment increases zinc excretion by as much as 60%, and supplementation is recommended for long-term treatment [81].

The interaction between zinc deficiency and acne was first reported in 1977 when it was noted that acne improved in patients being treated with zinc for acrodermatitis enteropathica [82]. Shortly thereafter, Michaelsson showed lower plasma zinc levels in patients with acne [83]. Since then, numerous studies, many reviewed by Cervantes et al., have been conducted evaluating the efficacy of oral and topical zinc in the treatment of acne, most demonstrating good efficacy with minimal side effects [72].

Rationale for the Use in the Treatment of Acne

Zinc has a plethora of activities that suggests a sound scientific rationale for its use in the treatment of acne. Its role in modulating immune response is eclectic, and it is involved in numerous inflammatory pathways thought to be important in acne pathogenesis, such as stimulation of natural killer cell and complement activity; inhibition of IL-6, TNF-alpha, and nitric oxide production; and integrin and toll-like receptor expression by keratinocytes [36, 84–89]. It has been shown to directly inhibit *C. acnes* proliferation and 5-alpha reductase, thereby suppressing sebaceous gland activity [36, 84, 89, 90].

Clinical Evidence of Zinc Efficacy in Acne

Cervantes evaluated 31 original studies and 1 case report evaluating the use of zinc, orally or topically, in the treatment of humans with at least mild acne. They found 12 studies in which zinc was used as monotherapy (11 oral and 1 topical) [91–102].

Six studies utilized combination therapy [59, 102–106] and 14 studies compared the zinc product to existing acne therapy [107–120]. Combinations included topical zinc with erythromycin and oral zinc in combination with nicotinamide and other vitamins and minerals. Comparative studies evaluated primarily oral zinc and oral antibiotics but also included topical zinc compared to clindamycin and erythromycin.

Overall, single-agent and combination studies suggested that zinc is an effective treatment option. However, comparative studies showed conflicting results. Zinc was found to be as effective or less effective than oral tetracycline and less effective than oral minocycline. Compared to erythromycin and clindamycin, studies suggest zinc may have equal or superior efficacy. Two findings are particularly noteworthy: one study found that zinc decreased facial "oiliness" in 58.6% of individuals compared to 0.0% in the lactose placebo arm [72]. In addition, a retrospective review found zinc, specifically zinc gluconate 75 mg daily (10 mg elemental zinc), to be safe during pregnancy [121].

Collectively these studies assessed effectiveness in 2356 patients. However, there were inconsistencies in dosing schedules, zinc formulations, and study endpoints, as well as significance of findings. Furthermore, less than half of the studies were controlled, making overall assessment of zinc efficacy and safety difficult. Many studies were short in duration—considerably shorter than FDA-mandated phase 3 pivotal trials for prescription drugs—and this may have falsely underestimated zinc overall efficacy.

Tolerability across all studies was good. Eleven of the 32 studies had at least 1 related adverse event—most commonly gastrointestinal symptoms such as nausea with oral agents—and cutaneous irritation with topical agents.

Evaluating the entirety of the zinc literature, it is undeniable that zinc is an inexpensive agent with a long safety track record, minimal side effects, and an extensive repertoire of plausible scientific rationales for its use in acne. Both in oral and topical formulations, most studies suggest clinical efficacy. However, larger controlled and double-blinded studies need to be conducted to better determine appropriate treatment regimens.

Miscellaneous

Sulfur

Sulfur has been used to treat numerous cutaneous disorders, including acne since the mid-1950s. It is reduced to hydrogen sulfide within keratinocytes and is thought to break down keratin in the skin, resulting in comedolytic activity. It may also have activity against *C. acnes* [122]. While most often used clinically as a 5% preparation in combination with sodium sulfacetamide, its use is limited by its distinctive, pungent odor [123].

Chromium

Chromium is an essential trace element that is poorly understood. It is thought to affect insulin activity and is believed to improve glucose tolerance, enhance insulin sensitivity, and regulate protein, carbohydrate, and lipid metabolism.

Although it has not been studied in acne per se, two studies have evaluated chromium supplementation in patients with polycystic ovarian syndrome (PCOS), in which acne may be an associated finding [124, 125]. In one study, 35 girls with PCOS were given 1000 μg chromium picolinate daily for 6 months [124]. They noted a significant reduction in free testosterone and an improvement in menstrual irregularities but no change in hirsutism or acne. In contrast, a controlled study of 60 women with PCOS given 200 μg daily vs. placebo for 8 weeks showed beneficial effects on acne, hirsutism, and C-reactive protein levels [125].

Selenium

Selenium is an essential trace mineral that has anti-inflammatory and antioxidant activities. It is a component of glutathione peroxidase, whose main biological role is to protect against oxidative damage. It is thought to play a role in fertility and cognitive functioning. There is insufficient evidence to suggest that supplementation is of use in preventing human disease.

Like chromium, selenium supplementation has been evaluated in patients with PCOS in regard to its effects on reproductive outcomes, biomarkers of inflammation, and oxidative stress. In a double-blind, randomized, placebo-controlled trial, 64 women with PCOS received either 200 μg of selenium daily or placebo for 8 weeks [126]. Pregnancy rate in the selenium group was higher, serum dehydroepiandrosterone (DHEA) levels and C-reactive protein were reduced, and alopecia ($p = 0.004$) and acne ($p = 0.003$) had both improved. It is unknown if acne would improve in subjects without PCOS.

Clay Minerals

Clay washes, masks, and scrubs have become increasingly popular in recent years. Clay includes various combinations of kaolinite, palygorskite, smectites, and talc. Content varies greatly depending on the source. Applied as a face mask, clay has been shown to stimulate sebaceous secretions, remove surface oils, and inhibit the grown of *S. epidermidis* and *C. acnes* [127, 128]. Dead Sea mud was shown to inhibit the growth of *C. acnes* on agar plates [129]. One clinical trial evaluating the efficacy of a clay and jojoba oil mask in mild acne showed a 54% mean reduction in total lesion count in 192 subjects treated with mask 2 to 3 times per week for 6 weeks [130]. More data, including a randomized double-blinded study, is necessary for adequate evaluation of clay in the treatment of acne.

Conclusion

Definitive data (with the exception of synthetic vitamin A topicals and orals) proving the efficacy of vitamins and minerals in the treatment of acne are lacking. However, there exists sound scientific rationale, considerable in vitro data, and increasingly convincing in vivo data indicating the usefulness of nicotinamide and zinc in acne. Vitamins D and C are more theoretical, and vitamin E and clay minerals have a paucity of data to support their use. Supplemental vitamin B12 may exacerbate acne severity. Chromium and selenium supplementation has data limited to patients with PCOS.

It is possible that combinations of vitamins and minerals will prove to be more efficacious than monotherapy, but data, again, is lacking. Fortunately, while waiting for more definitive data, we can afford to be generous with our recommendations with these agents, since as long as we stay within safety limitations, there is no harm to polytherapy.

References

1. Thielitz A, Gollnick H. Topical retinoids in acne vulgaris: update on efficacy and safety. Am J Clin Dermatol. 2008;9(6):369–81.
2. Czernielewski J, Michel S. Adapalene biochemistry and the evolution of a new topical retinoid for treatment of acne. J Eur Acad Dermatol Venereol. 2001;15(Suppl 3):5–12.
3. Tenaud I, Khammari A. In vitro modulation of TLR-2, CD1d and IL-10 by adapalene on normal human skin and acne inflammatory lesions. Exp Dermatol. 2007;16:500–6.
4. Olson J, Shah N. Vitamin A toxicity. Available at: www.ncbi.nlm.nih.gov. Accessed 4 December 2019.
5. Hunt J. Teratogenicity of high vitamin A intake. N Engl J Med. 1996;334(18):1197.
6. Vanchinathan V, Lim H. A dermatologist's perspective on vitamin D. Mayo Clin Proc. 2012;87:372–80.
7. Mostafa WZ, Hegazy RA. Vitamin D and the skin: focus on a complex relationship: a review. J Adv Res. 2015;6(6):793–804.
8. Amson Y, Amital H, Shoenfeld Y. Vitamin D and autoimmunity: new aetiological and therapeutic considerations. Ann Rheum Dis. 2007;66:1137–42.
9. Kostoglou-Athanassious I, Athanassious P, Lyraki A, Raftakis I, Antoniadis C. Vitamin D and rheumatoid arthritis. Ther Adv Endocrinol Metab. 2012;3:181–7.
10. Cheng H, Kim S, Park G, Chang SE, Bang S, Won CH, et al. Low vitamin D levels are associated with atopic dermatitis, but not allergic rhinitis, asthma, or IgE sensitization, in the adult Korean population. J Allergy Clin Immunol. 2014;133:1048–55.
11. Gisondi P, Rossini M, Di Cesare A, Idolazzi L, Farina S, Beltrami G, et al. Vitamin D status in patients with chronic plaque psoriasis. Br J Dermatol. 2012;166:505–10.

12. Silverberg JI, Silverberg AI, Malka E, Silverberg NB. A pilot study assessing the role of 25 hydroxy vitamin D levels in patients with vitiligo vulgaris. J Am Acad Dermatol. 2010;62:937–41.
13. Aksu Cerman A, Sarikaya Solak S, Kivanc AI. Vitamin D deficiency in alopecia areata. Br J Dermatol. 2014;170:1299–304.
14. Agak GW, Qin M, Nobe J, Kim MH, Krutzik SR, Tristan GR, et al. Propionibacterium acnes induces an IL-17 response in acne vulgaris that is regulated by Vitamin A and Vitamin D. J Invest Dermatol. 2014;134:366–73.
15. Reichrath J, Schuler C, Seifert M, et al. The vitamin D endocrine system of human sebocytes. Exp Dermatol. 28 June 2008. Available at: https://onlinelibrary.wiley.com/doi/abs/10.1111/j.1600-0625.2006.00439b.x.
16. Schauber J, Dorschner RA, Coda AB, Büchau AS, Liu PT, Kiken D, et al. Injury enhances TLR2 function and antimicrobial peptide expression through a vitamin D-dependent mechanism. J Clin Invest. 2007;117:803–11.
17. Lee WJ, Choi YH, Sohn MY, Lee SJ, Kim DW. Expression of inflammatory biomarkers from cultured sebocytes was influenced by treatment with vitamin D. Indian J Dermatol. 2013;58:327.
18. Lim SK, Ha JM, Lee Y, Lee Y, Seo YJ, Kim CD, et al. Comparison of vitamin D levels in patients with and without acne: a case-control study combined with a randomized controlled trial. PLoS One. 2016;11(8):e0161162.
19. Stewart T, Bazergy C. Hormonal and dietary factors in acne vulgaris vs. controls. Dermatoendocrinol. 2018;10(1):e1442160.
20. Yildizgoren M, Togral A. Preliminary evidence for vitamin D deficiency in nodulocystic acne vulgaris. Dermatoendocrinol. 2014;6(1):e983687.
21. Toossi P, Azizian Z, Yavari H, Fakhim TH, Amini SH, Enamzade R. Serum 25-hydroxy vitamin D levels in patients with acne vulgaris and its association with disease severity. Clin Cases Miner Bone Metab. 2015;12(3):238–42.
22. Al-Taiar A, AlKabbaz M, Rahman A, Al-Sabah R, Shaban L, Akhtar S. Plasma 25-hydroxy vitamin D is not associated with acne vulgaris. Nutrients. 2018;10(10):E1525.
23. Jarosz A, El-Sohemy A. Association between vitamin D status and premenstrual syndrome. J Acad Nutr Diet. 2019;119(1):115–23.
24. Lee WJ, Kim SL, Choe YS, Jang YH, Lee SJ, Kim DW. Magnesium ascorbyl phosphate regulates the expression of inflammatory biomarkers in cultured sebocytes. Ann Dermatol. 2015;27(4):376–82.

25. Nusgens BV, Humbert P, Rougier A, Colige AC, Haftek M, Lambert CA, et al. Topically applied vitamin C enhances the mRNA level of collagens I and III, their processing enzymes and tissue inhibitor of matrix metalloproteinase 1 in the human dermis. J Invest Dermatol. 2001;116:853–9.
26. Farue M, Kadano T. Inflammatory skin march in atopic dermatitis and psoriasis. Inflamm Res. 2017;66(10):838–42.
27. Yamamoto A, Takenovichi K, Ito M. Impaired water barrier function in acne vulgaris. Arch Dermatol Res. 1995;287:214–8.
28. Liu J, Yan R, Zhong Q, Ngo S, Bangayan NJ, Nguyen L, et al. The diversity and host interactions of Propionibacterium acnes bacteriophages on human skin. ISME J. 2015;9(9):2078–93.
29. Coughlin CC, Swink SM, Horwinski J, Sfyroera G, Bugayev J, Grice EA, et al. The preadolescent acne microbiome: a prospective, randomized, pilot study investigating characterization and effects of acne therapy. Pediatr Dermatol. 2017;34(6):661–4.
30. Kelhala HL, Aho VTE, Fyhrquist N, Pereira PAB, Kubin ME, Paulin L, et al. Isotretinoin and lymecycline treatments modify the skin microbiota in acne. Exp Dermatol. 2018;27(1):30–6.
31. McCoy WH 4th, Otchere E, Rosa BA, Martin J, Mann CM, Mitreva M. Skin ecology during sebaceous drought. How skin microbes respond to isotretinoin. J Invest Dermatol. 2019;139:732–5.
32. Shin J, Kim YJ, Kwon O, Kim NI, Cho Y. Associations among plasma vitamin C, epidermal ceramide and clinical severity of atopic dermatitis. Nutr Res Pract. 2016;10:398–403.
33. Khan H, Akhtar N, Ali A. Assessment of compound ascorbyl palmitate (AD) and sodium ascorbyl phosphate (SAP) on facial skin sebum control in female healthy volunteers. Drug Res (Stuttg). 2017;67(1):52–8.
34. Pinnell S. Cutaneous photodamage, oxidative stress and topical antioxidant protection. J Am Acad Dermatol. 2003;48:1–22.
35. Kosari P, Alikhan A, Sockolov M, Feldman SR. Vitamin E and allergic contact dermatitis. Dermatitis. 2010;21(3):148–53.
36. Ozuguz P, Dogruk Kacar S, Ekiz O, Takci Z, Balta I, Kalkan G. Evaluation of serum vitamins A and E and zinc levels according to the severity of acne vulgaris. Cutan Ocul Toxicol. 2014;33(2):99–102.
37. Valacchi G, Rimbach G, Salion C, et al. Effect of benzoyl peroxide on antioxidant status, NF-kappaB activity and interleukin-1alpha gene expression in human keratinocytes. Toxicology. 2001;165(2–3):22–34.

38. Rota C, Tomasi A, Iannone A. Alpha-tocopherol amplifies benzoyl peroxide free radical decomposition in a chemical system. Free Radic Res. 2006;40(6):637–45.
39. Knip M, Douek IF, Moore WP, Gillmor HA, McLean AE, Bingley PJ, et al. Safety of high-dose nicotinamide: a review. Diabetologia. 2000;43:1337–45.
40. Fisher GJ, Kang S, Varani J, Bata-Csorgo Z, Wan Y, Datta S, et al. Mechanisms of photoaging and chronological skin aging. Arch Dermatol. 2002;138(11):1462–70.
41. Namazi MR. Nicotinamide: a potential addition to the antipsoriatic weaponry. FASEB J. 2003;17(11):1377–9.
42. Fivenson DP, Breneman DL, Rosen GB, Hersh CS, Cardone S, Mutasim D. Nicotinamide and tetracycline therapy of bullous pemphigoid. Arch Dermatol. 1994;130(6):753–8.
43. Navarette-Solis J, Castanedo-Cazaras J, Torres-Alvarez B, et al. A double-blind, randomized clinical trial of niacinamide 4% versus hydroquinone 4% in the treatment of melasma. Dermatol Res Pract. 2011;379173:2011.
44. Chen AC, Martin AJ, Choy B, Fernández-Peñas P, Dalziell RA, McKenzie CA, et al. A phase 3 randomized trial of nicotinamide for skin-cancer chemoprevention. N Engl J Med. 2015;373(17):1618–26.
45. Grange PA, Raingeaud J, Calvez V, Dupin N. Nicotinamide inhibits Propionibacterium acnes-induced IL-8 production in keratinocytes through the NF-kappaB and MAPK pathways. J Dermatol Sci. 2009;56:106–12.
46. Wohlrab J, Kreft D. Niacinamide – mechanisms of action and its topical use in dermatology. Skin Pharmacol Physiol. 2014;27:311–5.
47. Draelos Z, Matsubara A, Smiles K. The effect of 2% niacinamide on facial sebum production. J Cosmet Laser Ther. 2006;8:96–101.
48. Fivenson DP. The mechanisms of action of nicotinamide and zinc in inflammatory skin disease. Cutis. 2006;77:5–10.
49. Walocko FM, Eber AE, Keri JE, Al-Harbi MA, Nouri K. The role of nicotinamide in acne treatment. Dermatol Ther. 2017;30(5):e12481. https://doi.org/10.1111/dth.12481. Epub 2017 Feb 21.
50. Khodaeiani E, Fouladi RF, Amirnia M, Saeidi M, Karimi ER. Topical 4% nicotinamide vs. 1% clindamycin in moderate inflammatory acne vulgaris. Int J Dermatol. 2013;52:999–1004.
51. Shahmoradi Z, Iragi F, Siadat AH, Ghorbaini A. Comparison of topical 5% nicotinamide gel versus 2% clindamycin gel in the

treatment of the mild-moderate acne vulgaris: a double-blinded randomized clinical trial. J Res Med Sci. 2013;18:115–7.
52. Shalita AR, Smith JG, Parish LC, Sofman MS, Chalker DK. Topical nicotinamide compared with clindamycin gel in the treatment of inflammatory acne vulgaris. Int J Dermatol. 1995;34:434–7.
53. Kaymak Y, Onder M. An investigation of efficacy of topical niacinamide for the treatment of mild and moderate acne vulgaris. J Turk Acad Dermatol. 2008;2(4):jtad82402a. Available at: http://www.jtad.org/2008/4/jtad82402a.pdf.
54. Dos SK, Barbhuiya JN, Jana S, Dey SK. Comparative evaluation of clindamycin phosphate 1% and clindamycin phosphate 1% with nicotinamide gel 4% in the treatment of acne vulgaris. Indian J Dermatol Venereol Leprol. 2003;69:8–9.
55. Sardesai V, Kambli V. Comparison of efficacy of topical clindamycin and nicotinamide combination with plain clindamycin for the treatment of acne vulgaris and acne resistant to topical antibiotics. Indian J Dermatol Venereol Leprol. 2003;69:138–9.
56. Morganti P, Berardesca E, Guarneri B, Guarneri F, Fabrizi G, Palombo P, et al. Topical clindamycin 1% vs linoleic acid-rich phosphatidylcholine and nicotinamide 4% in the treatment of acne: a multicentre-randomized trial. Int J Cosmet Sci. 2011;33:467–76.
57. Emanuele E, Bertona M, Altabas K, Altabas V, Alessandrini G. Anti-inflammatory effects of topical preparation containing nicotinamide, retinol, and 7-dehydrocholesterol in patients with acne: a gene expression study. Clin Cosmet Investig Dermatol. 2012;5:33–7.
58. Niren N, Torok H. The nicomide improvement inclinical outcomes study (NICOS): results of an 8-week trial. Cutis. 2006;77:17–28.
59. Shalita AR, Falcon R, Olansky A, Iannotta P, Akhavan A, Day D, et al. Inflammatory acne management with a novel prescription dietary supplement. J Drugs Dermatol. 2012;11:1428–33.
60. Jadassohn W, Paillard R, Hofer R, et al. Vitamin B12 et poussee aceneiforme. Dermatologica. 1958;116:349. In French.
61. Puissant A, Vanbremeersch F, Monfort J, Lamberton JN. A new iatrogenic dermatosis: acne caused by vitamin B 12. Bull Soc Fr Dermatol Syphiligr. 1967;74:813–5. In French.
62. Braun-Falco O, Lincke H. The problem of vitamin B6/B12 acne. A contribution on acne medicamentosa (author's transl). MMW Munch Med Wochenschr. 1976;118:155–60. In German.

63. Dupre A, Albarel N, Bonafe JL, Christol B, Lassere J. Vitamin B-12 induced acnes. Cutis. 1979;24:210–1.
64. Sherertz E. Acneiform eruption due to "megadose" vitamins B6 and B12. Cutis. 1991;48:119.
65. Balta I, Ozuguz P. Vitamin B12-induced acneiform eruption. Cutan Ocul Toxicol. 2014;33:94–5.
66. Goldblatt S. Vitamin B-12 levels in blood serum in acne-like skin diseases. Hautarzt. 1966;17:106–8. In German.
67. Karadag AS, Tutal E, Ertugrul DT, Akin KO. Effect of isotretinoin treatment on plasma holotranscobalamin, vitamin B12, folic acid, and homocysteine levels: non-controlled study. Int J Dermatol. 2011;50:1564–9.
68. Kang D, Shi B, Erfe MC, Craft N, Li H. Vitamin B12 modulates the transcriptome of the skin microbiota in acne pathogenesis. Sci Transl Med. 2015;7(293):293ra103.
69. Sharma CM, Hoffmann S, Darfeuille F, Reignier J, Findeiss S, Sittka A, et al. The primary transcriptome for the major human pathogen Helicobacter pylori. Nature. 2010;464:250–5.
70. Lundrigan M, Kadner R. Altered cobalamin metabolism in Escherichia coli btuR mutants affects btuB gene regulation. J Bacteriol. 1989;171:154–61.
71. Piomelli S, Davidow B, Guinee VF, Young P, Gay G. The FEP (free erythrocyte porphyrins) test: a screening micromethod for lead poisoning. Pediatrics. 1973;51:254–9.
72. Cervantes J, Eber AE, Perper M, Nascimento VM, Nouri K, Keri JE. The role of zinc in the treatment of acne: a review of the literature. Dermatol Ther. 2018;31(1):e12576. https://doi.org/10.1111/dth.12576.
73. Sanstead H. Understanding zinc: recent observations and interpretation. J Lab Clin Med. 1994;124:322–7.
74. Solomons N. Mild human zinc deficiency produces an imbalance between cell-mediated and humoral immunity. Nutr Rev. 1998;56:27–8.
75. Prasad A. Zinc: an overview. Nutrition. 1995;11:93–9.
76. Broun ER, Greist A, Tricot G, Hoffman R. Excessive zinc ingestion. A reversible cause of sideroblastic anemia and bone marrow depression. JAMA. 1990;264:1441–3.
77. Willis MS, Monaghan SA, Miller ML, McKenna RW, Perkins WD, Levinson BS, et al. Zinc-induced copper deficiency: a report of three cases initially recognized on bone marrow examination. Am J Clin Pathol. 2005;123:125–31.

78. Duncan A, Yacoubian C, Watson N, Morrison I. The risk of copper deficiency in patients prescribed zinc supplements. J Clin Pathol. 2015;68(9):723–5.
79. Lomaestro B, Bailae G. Absorption interactions with fluoroquinolones. 1995 update. Drug Saf. 1995;12:314–33.
80. Penttila O, Hurme H, Neuvonen P. Effect of zinc sulfate on the absorption of tetracycline and doxycycline in man. Eur J Clin Pharmacol. 1975;9:131–4.
81. Webster P. Urinary zinc excretion during treatment with different diuretics. Acta Med Scand. 1980;208:209–12.
82. Fitzherbert J. Zinc deficiency in acne vulgaris. Med J Aust. 1977;2:685–6.
83. Michaelsson G, Vahlquist A, Juhlin L. Serum zinc and retinol-binding protein in acne. Br J Dermatol. 1977;96:283–6.
84. Azzouni F, Godoy A, Li Y, Mohler J. The 5 alpha-reductase isozyme family: a review of basic biology and their role in human diseases. Adv Urol. 2012;2012:530121.
85. Chow SC. Immunomodulation by statins: mechanisms and potential impact on autoimmune diseases. Arch Immunol Ther Exp. 2009;57:243–51.
86. Gupta M, Mahajan VK, Mehta KS, Chauhan PS. Zinc therapy in dermatology: a review. Dermatol Res Pract. 2014;2014:709152.
87. Kitamura H, Morikawa H, Kamon H, Iguchi M, Hojyo S, Fukada T, et al. Toll-like receptor-mediated regulation of zinc homeostasis influences dendritic cell function. Nat Immunol. 2006;7:971–7.
88. Sardana K, Chugh S, Garg V. The role of zinc in acne and prevention or resistance: have we missed the "base" effects. Int J Dermatol. 2014;53:125–7.
89. Sugimoto Y, Lopez-Solache I, Labrie F, Luu-The V. Cations inhibit specifically type 1 5 alpha-reductase found in human skin. J Invest Dermatol. 1995;104:775–8.
90. Bae J, Park S. Evaluation of antimicrobial activity of zinc oxide, citric acid and a mix of both against Propionibacterium acnes. Int J Cosmet Sci. 2016;38(6):550–7.
91. Cochran R, Tucker S, Flannigan S. Topical zinc therapy for acne vulgaris. Int J Dermatol. 1985;24:188–90.
92. Dreno B, Amblard P, Agache P, Sirot S, Litoux P. Low doses of zinc gluconate for inflammatory acne. Acta Derm Venereol. 1989;69:541–3.
93. Dreno B, Floulc P, Reynaud A, Moyse D, Habert H, Richet H. Effect of zinc gluconate on propionibacterium acnes resistance to erythromycin in patients with inflammatory acne: in vitro and in vivo study. Eur J Dermatol. 2005;15:152–5.

94. Goransson K, Liden S, Odsell L. Oral zinc in acne vulgaris: a clinical and methodological study. Acta Derm Venereol. 1978;58:443–8.
95. Hillström L, Pettersson L, Hellbe L, Kjellin A, Leczinsky CG, Nordwall C. Comparison of oral treatment with zinc sulfate and placebo in acne vulgaris. Br J Dermatol. 1977;97:681–4.
96. Kobayashi H, Aiba S, Tagami H. Successful treatment of dissecting cellulitis and acne conglobate with oral zinc. Br J Dermatol. 1999;141:1137–8.
97. Meynadier J. Efficacy and safety study of two zinc gluconate regiments in the treatment of inflammatory acne. Eur J Dermatol. 2000;10:269–73.
98. Orris L, Shalita A, Sibulkin D, London SJ, Gans EH. Oral zinc therapy of acne. Absorption and clinical effect. Arch Dermatol. 1978;114:1018–20.
99. Verma K, Saini A, Dhamija S. Oral zinc sulphate therapy in acne vulgaris: a double-blind trial. Acta Derm Venereol. 1980;60:337–40.
100. Weimar VM, Puhl SC, Smith WH, tenBroeke JE. Xinc sulfate in acne vulgaris. Arch Dermatol. 1978;114:1776–8.
101. Weismann K, Wadskov S, Sondergaard J. Oral zinc sulphate therapy for acne vulgaris. Acta Derm Venereol. 1977;57:357–60.
102. Capitanio B, Sinagra JL, Weller RB, Brown C, Berardesca E. Randomized controlled study of a cosmetic treatment for mild acne. Clin Exp Dermatol. 2012;37:346–9.
103. Fluhr JW, Bosch B, Gloor M, Höffler U. In-vitro and in-vivo efficacy of zinc acetate against propionibacteria alone and in combination with erythromycin. Zentralbl Bakteriol. 1999;289:445–56.
104. Sardana K, Garg V. An observational study of methionine-bound zinc with antioxidants for mild to moderate acne vulgaris. Dermatol Ther. 2010;23:411–8.
105. Schachner L, Eaglstein W, Kittles C, Mertz P. Topical erythromycin and zinc therapy for acne. J Am Acad Dermatol. 1990;22:253–60.
106. Strauss JS, Stranieri AM. Acne treatment with topical erythromycin and zinc: effect of propionibacterium acnes and free fatty acid composition. J Am Acad Dermatol. 1984;11:86–9.
107. Bojar RA, Eady EA, Jones CE, Cunliffe WJ, Holland KT. Inhibition of erythromycin-resistant propionibacteria on the skin of acne patients by topical erythromycin with and without zinc. Br J Dermatol. 1994;130:329–36.

108. Chu A, Huber F, Plott R. The comparative efficacy of benzoyl peroxide 5%/erythromycin 3% gel and erythromycin 4%/zinc 1.2% solution in the treatment of acne vulgaris. Br J Dermatol. 1997;136:235–8.
109. Cunliffe WJ, Burke B, Dodman B, Gould DJ. A double-blind trial of a zinc sulphate/citrate complex and tetracycline in the treatment of acne vulgaris. Br J Dermatol. 1979;101:321–5.
110. Cunliffe WJ, Fernandez C, Bojar R, Kanis R, West F, Zindaclin Clinical Study Group. An observer-blind parallel-group, randomized, multicentre clinical and microbiological study of a topical clindamycin/zinc gel and a topical clindamycin lotion in patients with mild/moderate acne. J Dermatolog Treat. 2005;16:213–8.
111. Dreno B, Moyse D, Alirezai M, Amblard P, Auffret N, Beylot C, et al. Multicenter randomized comparative double-blind controlled clinical trial of the safety and efficacy of zinc gluconate versus minocycline hydrochloride in the treatment of inflammatory acne vulgaris. Dermatology. 2001;203:135–40.
112. Feucht CL, Allen BS, Chalker DK, Smith JG Jr. Topical erythromycin with zinc in acne. A double-blind controlled study. J Am Acad Dermatol. 1980;3:483–91.
113. Habbema L, Koopmans B, Menke HE, Doornweerd S, De Boulle K. A 4% erythromycin and zinc combination (Zineryt) versus 2% erythromycin (Eryderm) in acne vulgaris: a randomized, double-blind comparative study. Br J Dermatol. 1989;121(4):497–502.
114. Langner A, Sheehan-Dare R, Layton A. A randomized, single-blind comparison of topical clindamycin + benzoyl peroxide (Duac) and erythromycin + zinc acetate (Zineryt) in the treatment of mild to moderate facial acne vulgaris. J Eur Acad Dermatol Venereol. 2007;21:311–9.
115. Michaëlsson G. Oral zinc in acne. Acta Derm Venereol Suppl (Stockh). 1980;Suppl 89:87–93.
116. Michaëlsson G, Juhlin L, Ljunghall K. A double-blind study of the effect of zinc and oxytetracycline in acne vulgaris. Br J Dermatol. 1977;97:561–6.
117. Michaëlsson G, Juhlin L, Vahlquist A. Effects of oral zinc and vitamin A in acne. Arch Dermatol. 1977;113:31–6.
118. Papageorgious P, Chu A. Chloroxylenol and zinc oxide containing cream in the treatment of acne vulgaris. A double-bling randomized, controlled trial. Clin Exp Dermatol. 2000;113:31–6.
119. Schachner L, Pestana A, Kittles C. A clinical trial comparing the safety and efficacy of a topical erythromycin-zinc formulation

with a topical clindamycin formulations. J Am Acad Dermatol. 1990;22:489–95.
120. Sharquie KE, Noaimi AA, Al-Salih MM. Topical therapy of acne vulgaris using 2% tea lotion in comparison with 5% zinc sulphate solution. Saudi Med J. 2008;29:1757–61.
121. Dreno B, Blouin E. Acne, pregnant women and zinc salts: a literature review. Ann Dermatol Venereol. 2008;135(1):7–33.
122. Akhavan A, Bershad S. Topical acne drugs. Am J Clin Dermatol. 2003;4:473–92.
123. Del Rosso J. The use of sodium sulfacetamide 10%/sulfur 5% emollient foam in the treatment of acne. J Clin Aesthet Dermatol. 2009;2(8):26–9.
124. Amr N, Abdel-Rahim H. The effect of chromium supplementation on PCOS in adolescents. J Pediatr Adolesc Gynecol. 2015;28(2):114–8.
125. Jamilian M, Bahmani F, Siavashani MA, Mazloomi M, Asemi Z, Esmaillzadeh A. The effects of chromium supplementation on endocrine profiles, biomarkers of inflammation, and oxidative stress in women with polycystic ovary syndrome: a randomized, double blind, placebo-controlled trial. Biol Trace Elem Res. 2016;172(1):71–8.
126. Razavi M, Jamilian M, Kashan Z. Selenium supplementation and the effects on reproductive outcomes, biomarkers of inflammation, and oxidative stress in women with polycystic ovary syndrome. Horm Metab Res. 2016;48(3):185–90.
127. Carretero M. Clay minerals and their beneficial effect upon human health. A review. Appl Clay Sci. 2002;21:155–63.
128. Park S, Lee C, Lee M. Antibacterial effect of minerals from ores indigenous to Korea. J Environ Biol. 2009;30:151–4.
129. Ma'or Z, Henis Y, Alon Y, Orlov E, Sørensen KB, Oren A. Antimicrobial properties of Dead Sea black mineral mud. Int J Dermatol. 2006;45:504–11.
130. Meier L, Stange R, Michalsen A, Uehleke B. Clay jojoba oil facial mask for lesioned skin and mild acne – results of a prospective, observational pilot study. Forsch Komplementmed. 2012;19(2):75–9.

Chapter 3
Oral Botanical Supplements

Michal Solomon and Adriana Leite

Di-indolyl Methane

A diet rich in cruciferous vegetables such as cauliflower, broccoli, and cabbage has long been considered healthy, and various epidemiological studies suggest that the consumption of cruciferous vegetables contributes to a cancer-protecting diet.

Indole-3-carbinol (I3C) is derived from naturally occurring glucosinolates in cruciferous vegetables. It is rapidly converted into a range of metabolites under the acidic stomach environment, among which 3,3-diindolylmethane (DIM) is the most prominent compound [4]. DIM exerts several biological activities on cellular and molecular levels, which contribute to its well-recognized chemoprevention potential [5, 6].

DIM restores healthy hormone balance by adjusting the balance of bad estrogens to good estrogens, and it blocks aromatase, which converts testosterone to estrogen. Di-indolyl methane is used for preventing breast, uterine, and colorectal

M. Solomon (✉)
Department of Dermatology, Sheba Medical Center, Ramat Gan, Israel

A. Leite
Department of Dermatology, All Beauty Company, São Paulo, Brazil

R. N. Rupani, P. A. Lio (eds.), *Integrative Dermatology*,
https://doi.org/10.1007/978-3-030-58954-7_3

cancer. It is also used to prevent an enlarged prostate (benign prostatic hypertrophy, or BPH) and to treat premenstrual syndrome (PMS) and, apparently, hormonal acne. DIM is generally well tolerated, with a few mild symptoms lasting a few days. Side effects of DIM include headache, fatigue, brain fog, and dark urine (orange to brownish color).

Typically, DIM will come in 100–200 mg capsules. It is recommended to start slow, with 100 mg every day or every other day until you no longer have detox symptoms.

Vitex agnus-castus

Vitex agnus-castus (VAC)—also known as chaste tree, chasteberry, and monk's pepper—is a deciduous shrub that is native to the Mediterranean, Europe, and Central Asia. It has been used for female reproductive disorders since ancient Greek and Roman times. In the fourth century B.C., Hippocrates recommended the plant for injuries, inflammation, and swelling of the spleen. VAC is also mentioned in the works of Dioscorides and Theophrastus [7]. The name agnus-castus derives from the Latin words "castitas" (chastity) and "agnus" (lamb); it is also called chaste tree, which refers to its ability to decrease sexual desire and promote chastity in women and celibacy in monks. Another common name, monk's pepper, originates from its use by monks as a spice in cooking.

Traditionally, VAC has been used by practitioners of phytotherapy in the treatment of many female conditions, including menstrual disorders (amenorrhea, dysmenorrhea), premenstrual syndrome (PMS), corpus luteum insufficiency, hyperprolactinemia, infertility, acne, menopause, and disrupted lactation [8]. In popular medicine, VAC is also considered to be an emmenagogue, vulnerary, carminative, lactagogue, anthelmintic, and anti-inflammatory [9]. The German Commission E has approved the use of VAC for irregularities of the menstrual cycle, premenstrual disturbances, and mastodynia [10].

In Europe, the parts used for medicinal purposes are the ripe dried fruit and extracts/concentrates of this part of the plant. Its constituents are flavonoids (casticin, isovitexin, orientin), iridoids (aucubin, agnuside, eurostide), volatile oils (monoterpenes and sesquiterpenes), linoleic acid, and a bitter principle called castine [11, 12]. The whole plant extract is considered necessary for the therapeutic action [13].

VAC is believed to act on the hypothalamus and pituitary gland, thus indirectly altering the balance of sex hormones. The mode of action of VAC is not completely understood, and several mechanisms have been considered. The most probable is an interaction with dopaminergic receptors in the anterior pituitary gland, with a subsequent reduction of prolactin secretion, derived from evidence from human in vivo studies [14–16]. Prolactin is produced by the anterior pituitary gland and plays an important role in a variety of reproductive functions [17]; prolactin levels rise naturally during pregnancy to induce the development of the mammary glands and to stimulate milk production. Raised levels of prolactin in nonlactating women are associated with female disorders, such as cyclic breast tenderness, menstrual abnormalities, absence of ovulation, and some symptoms of PMS [17]. Other reviews are available for the efficacy of VAC in PMS, cycle disorders, hyperprolactinemia, and mastalgia [18].

Some side effects of *Vitex agnus-cactus* are minor dermal problems and some intestinal problems such as diarrhea, headache, vertigo, and palpitation, which disappear after stopping its use [19]. There are no reports of herb–drug interactions involving *Vitex agnus-cactus*. Some herbalists believe that *Vitex agnus-cactus* could interfere with birth control pills, hormone replacement therapy, and other hormone replacement medications [19]. Additionally, it has been hypothesized that individuals taking drugs classified as dopamine receptor antagonists should use *Vitex agnus-cactus* with caution because animal studies indicate that *Vitex agnus-cactus* may interfere with the dopamine receptors [20, 21].

Several studies have been done to evaluate the effects of *Vitex agnus-cactus* on PMS, and most of them have revealed its significant effects on decreasing or improving PMS symptoms [22–24].

Vitex agnus-castus has been used for acne before menstruation. The whole fruit extract acting on follicle stimulating and luteinizing hormone levels in the pituitary gland led to an increase in progesterone and decrease in estrogen levels through the dopaminergic mechanism, decreasing the level of premenstrual prolactin. The German Commission E has recommended daily intake of 40 mg of *Vitex agnus-castus* extract for the treatment of acne. Pregnant and nursing women should not use this plant. Adverse side effects such as gastrointestinal disturbances and skin rashes have been reported [25].

Adaptogens and the Skin

Adaptogenic herbs help modulate our response to stress [26]. Stress stimulates cortisol release, which drives skin oil production and increases pro-inflammatory cytokines, impairing skin barrier function, including the ability to retain water. Adaptogens have immune-potentiating activity mediated through the modulation of T-cell immunity [27].

The growing field of psychodermatology addresses the link between an emotional state and the body's physiological response. Recent research has confirmed the skin both as an immediate stress perceiver and as a target of stress responses [28]. Skin disorders such as acne and rosacea have a high impact on a patient's behavior and emotional state, which then leads to further stress signaling and a positive feedback loop.

The body response to stress-producing hormones like cortisol and its metabolic changes include inflammation, unbalanced oil production, and increased sensitivity. Sleep deprivation also increases cortisol levels, disrupting skin barrier function and homeostasis, leading to microbial imbalance. Clinically, this variably manifests as oiliness or dryness, dehydration, and redness.

Adaptogens can play a role in stabilizing emotional responses to environmental stressors, thereby normalizing physiological processes promoting homeostasis [3, 29, 30]. Some of the properties that adaptogens may bring are anti-anxiety, immune modulating, antimicrobial, and anti-inflammatory activities. Also the use of adaptogen-based preparations increases the nonspecific phase of stress resistance, facilitating the achievement and prolonged maintenance of allostasis [30].

Acne vulgaris affects about 85% of teenagers and may continue to adulthood. Acne is one of the most prevalent skin diseases. Acne is usually due to an increase in body androgens, hyperkeratinization, and skin microbiota imbalance and occurs more often in adolescence during puberty, but also can be present into adulthood [3].

Even though many conventional acne treatment options are available, they carry risks and mild to severe side effects, and none is completely satisfactory. This creates the opportunity for many herbal medicine studies and clinical trials to gain research support showing that it has many possibilities to offer clinically in this disorder.

Rosacea is an inflammatory disease that is erroneously termed "acne–rosacea" despite differing pathogenesis. Recent studies have found associations between rosacea and an increased risk of potentially serious systemic disorders [31]. A recent study found that rosacea patients had elevated levels of oxidative stress or an imbalance between free radicals and antioxidants in the blood [32, 33]. Comparing patient blood samples from 50 rosacea patients and 42 healthy control patients, it was found that rosacea patients had higher levels of disulfides and lower thiols than the control group.

Thiols are antioxidants produced by the body to neutralize free radicals. The neutralization process turns thiols into disulfides, and the ratio of thiols to disulfides into the bloodstream can indicate the level of oxidative stress caused by UV radiation, diet, and other lifestyle factors [33]. The thiol-associated antioxidant mechanisms may play a role in the inflammation of rosacea and suggest that antioxidant treatments might be an adjuvant therapy for rosacea [33].

Adaptogens can be useful in the treatment of both acne and rosacea, in that disease pathogenesis includes stress-induced inflammation [29].

CRH (corticotropin-releasing hormone) and its receptors have been detected on sebocytes [34]. It was shown that CRH promotes lipogenesis in sebocytes through upregulation of a key lipogenesis enzyme [34]. Stress also induces IL-6 and IL-11 cytokine production in keratinocytes, contributing to inflammation [34]. ACTH and alfa-MSH also contribute to sebum production and possibly worsen the acne phenotype [35, 36].

The role of neuropeptide, specifically substance P, in acne is well-known [35, 36]. Facial skin from acne patients shows marked increase of SP-positive nerve fibers around the sebaceous glands and around acne lesions [37]. SP induces gene expression of PPAR-gamma, which plays a unique role in stimulating sebocyte lipogenesis. Inflammatory responses induced by *Cutibacterium* acnes are a major etiological factor in the pathogenesis of acne vulgaris.

Those facts show that adaptogens can be an important adjuvant therapy in terms of helping to manage the stress and the resulting inflammatory cascade.

Pharmacological Action of Adaptogens

The mechanism of adaptogens is not possible to easily explain by using the reductionist concept of pharmacology [38]. Considering that the pharmacological activity of any phytochemical is not specific and associated only with one type of receptor, adaptogenic compounds affect key mediators of the adaptive stress response at both intracellular and extracellular levels of communication as described by Panossian [39]. Consequently, many molecular targets, signaling pathways, and networks are involved. Adaptogens may have antioxidant and anti-inflammatory properties and also act as lipogenesis modulators (lipostatic) and augment adaptations to noxious stimuli (exposure to cold, heat, pain, general stress, infectious organisms).

It is important to highlight that the origin and provenance of adaptogenic extracts need to be known, due to lack of standardization to guarantee authenticity and quality. We need to seek to know reliable suppliers to be able to reach the expected results when we recommend these high-value herbal medicine extracts. We need to avoid unregistered supplements aiming to establish real value chain. We need to enable patients and consumers to have confidence that the products are authentic and meet a high specification for quality and safety.

It is essential that we pay attention to bioavailability, standardization, and bio-optimization of these ingredients, as long as adaptogens are present at high concentrations in various plant species. The most popular ones that can be used for acne and rosacea treatments will be presented in this chapter.

Rhodiola rosea (Golden Root, Arctic Root, Rose Root)

Rhodiola is one of the most important medicinal herbs and belongs to plants revealing adaptogenic properties which are attributed to the presence of specific phenolic compounds and are mainly reflected as antioxidant activity. *R. rosea* also revealed strong antibacterial effects against, for example, *Staphylococcus* strains [40, 41]. Besides that, *Rhodiola rosea* has free radical scavenging activities by its oligomeric proanthocyanidin [41].

Among the chemical components of *Rhodiola* we have salidrosides, rosavins, tyrosol, polysaccharides, flavonoids, terpenoids, proanthocyanidins, flavonolignans, and others. Salidroside is the main bioactive agent. Approximately 200 chemical compounds have been isolated from *Rhodiola* species [40, 41].

Rosavins are known as phenylpropanoids (cinnamyl alcohol glycoside) which include rosavins, rosins, and rosarins. They are specific for *R. rosea* and not detected at other *Rhodiola* species [41–45]. Their mechanism of action remains unclear but must be combined with other, more powerful, compounds such as salidroside to enhance its properties.

Salidroside is a glucoside form of tyrosol. Studies have shown that one of the main mechanisms of action is by blocking monoamine oxidase enzymes. Those enzymes bind to the outer membrane of mitochondria, causing oxidative breakdown of various components and neurotransmitters, including dopamine, serotonin, and norepinephrine. Rhodiola may potentially lead to a significant increase of these neurotransmitters and also has potential to regulate cortisol.

It is important to know that there are more than 200 species of *Rhodiola*, of which approximately 20 are used as traditional medicine, mainly in Asia and Europe. Some species of *Rhodiola* and the species that come from China and Tibet as *Rhodiola crenulata* do not contain rosavins, but have high concentrations of salidrosides and p-tyrosol.

Rhodiola has therapeutic value for many diseases, due to its pharmacological functions and therapeutic actions. It is usually taken in the morning because it can be a stimulant.

The proportion between salidrosides and rosavins (this one present only in *Rhodiola rosea*) varies depending from the origin, so there is not a standard pattern.

Adaptogens in general should not be used by pregnant or nursing women because of lack of reliable studies. They also must not be combined with psychiatric medications as mood stabilizers without evaluating the interactions with some other medications (e.g., fluoxetine, paroxetine, and sertraline) due to the potential for cytochrome P450 2C9–CYP2C9 interactions.

Schisandra chinensis (Chinese Magnolia Vine, Wuweizi—"Five-Flavor Berry")

Schisandra chinensis is known as "five-flavor-fruit" because it possesses all five basic flavors. It comes from northern China and the Russian Far East, where it is considered as one of the 50 fundamental herbs. *Schisandra chinensis* extract has been shown in some studies to promote healthy stress levels, as it can decrease corticosteroids by increasing acetylcholine levels, and also can enhance cholinergic signaling. *Schisandra chinensis* contains many lignans including schisandrin types A, B, and C, as well as schisandrol A and B. In vitro tests have shown that schisandrins A, B, and C inhibit the release of inflammatory cytokines, decrease the levels of toll-like receptor 2 and schisandrin B and C, and reduce the intracellular mRNA expression of the receptor gene. It is known that innate immune response in acne vulgaris is related to activation of toll-like receptor 2 in inflammatory cytokine responses [46]. Furthermore, the three lignans also prevented the nuclear translocation of NF-kappaB [47, 48]. The extract must contain a minimum of 3% schisandrins to be effective.

It has been reported that schisandra possesses a variety of pharmacological activities against respiratory, gastrointestinal, neurological, cardiovascular, hepatic, and dermatologic diseases involving inflammatory pathways such as atopic dermatitis, acne, and rosacea, as described above [48]. Moreover, schisandrin B can protect the skin against solar irradiation-induced oxidative stress [49], protecting UVB-exposed fibroblasts from photoaging [50]. Furthermore, new studies revealed the anti-inflammatory and antibacterial effects of this herbal extract to control acne induced by *C. acnes*, suggesting that schisandrins might be developed as pharmacological agents for acne therapy [46, 48]. The study by Guo et al., conducted in vitro, found that schisandra significantly reduced pro-inflammatory cytokine levels of *C. acne*, stimulating levels of IL-8, IL-1beta, and TNF-alfa [48].

Schisandrins can block the inflammatory response and prevent *C. acnes* bacterial growth. This way, it would be very helpful besides the conventional acne therapies that are focused to reduce *C. acnes* density, as it is recognized as an important part in acne pathophysiology [48].

Ashwagandha (Withania somnifera, Indian Ginseng, Wild Cherry)

Ashwagandha is a small plant native to India, the Middle East, and parts of Africa. Its roots, leaves, and fruits are used in

Ayurvedic medicine to build resistance to stress, enhance mediated immunity, and protect from free radical damage. This herb is abundant in antioxidant, immune-boosting, antistress, sleep-inducing, anti-inflammatory, and antibacterial properties.

Ashwagandha contains steroidal lactones (withanolides) and other alkaloids like somniferine, sominine, and anferine that can mimic certain corticosteroids, interact with steroid receptors, modulate cortisol levels, and improve stress responses [51]. It can also decrease markers of inflammation such as CRP (C-reactive protein) and reduce LDC-C (low-density lipoprotein cholesterol), due to its hypolipidemic properties. It also contains iron, tannins, nitrates, potassium, glucose, fatty acids, flavonoids, and acyl steryl glucosides.

Withanolides have antioxidant and anti-inflammatory properties that help inhibit the growth of *Staphylococcus* bacteria [28]. Individuals with autoimmune diseases such as lupus, rheumatoid arthritis, type 1 diabetes, and Hashimoto's disease may need to avoid it, since ashwagandha can have an effect on blood sugar, inflammation, and hormone regulation. Ashwagandha root extract may stimulate activity in thyroid glands, which could be interesting to individuals suffering from subclinical hypothyroidism—which occurs in 3–8% of the global population—but its use must be always monitored by a doctor.

Ashwagandha is part of the nightshade family (Solanaceae), and some people could have an allergy or intolerance to it.

It is important to understand there are not enough long-term studies determining the appropriate oral dosage for ashwagandha. This depends on the patient's age, health, and purpose for use.

Ashwagandha also should not be used during pregnancy and breastfeeding, or combined with other medications like mood regulators, without medical advice.

Cannabidiol (*Cannabis sativa*, CBD)

CBD is a non-psychotropic, non-intoxicating phytocannabinoid of *Cannabis sativa* and is being hailed for its ability to balance the endocannabinoid system (ECS). It is through this process that it allows the body to handle stress, and it acts as an adaptogen. CBD works by two receptors in the ECS, CB-1 and CB-2, to help regulate sleep, mood, anxiety, and depression, lower stress levels, and normalize the immune system.

The ECS regulates multiple physiological processes, including cell growth and differentiation. Recently, it was shown that CBD behaves as a highly effective sebostatic agent, inhibiting the lipogenic actions of various compounds, including arachidonic acid, and a combination of linoleic acid and testosterone and suppressed sebocyte proliferation via TRPV-4 (transient potential receptor vanilloid-4) ion channels used in cultured human sebocytes and human skin organ culture [52, 53].

CBD also has anti-inflammatory and anti-proliferative effects, becoming a promising therapeutic agent for the treatment of acne.

Oláh A et al. showed in their studies that CBD demonstrated complex anti-acne effects by normalizing "pro-acne agents" as a unique "trinity of cellular anti-acne actions." They described that CBD primarily normalized the pathologically elevated lipogenesis induced by "pro-acne" agents, both in a quantitative and qualitative manner (universal lipostatic effect). Moreover, it suppresses cell proliferation (anti-proliferative effect) and also prevents the actions of TLR (keratinocyte toll-like receptors) activation or "pro-acne" agents to elevate pro-inflammatory cytokine levels (universal anti-inflammatory effect) [52, 53].

The exact pharmacokinetics of CBD by its systemic application in the human body is still unknown. Topical CBD administration, using appropriate vehicles, due its high lipophilicity, is expected to preferentially enter the skin via the transfollicular route to accumulate in the sebaceous glands [52, 53].

One of the phytocannabinoid substances, the non-psychotropic phytocannabinoid THCV (delta-9-tetrahydrocannabivarin), downregulated basal sebaceous lipid synthesis and might become highly efficient as a novel anti-acne agent [39, 52]. Further studies are warranted to determine the significance of these findings in the clinical setting, even though it seems to be very promising.

Turmeric (*Curcuma longa*, Indian Saffron, Golden Spice)

Turmeric is a spice widely used in Asia that comes from the root of *Curcuma longa*, and it has curcumin as its main ingredient (2–8%) besides other curcuminoids like demethoxycurcumin and bisdemethoxycurcumin. Curcumin is also known as diferuloylmethane. Although turmeric has been used for a long time in alternative medicine, curcumin has yet to merge as a component of our mainstream dermatologic therapeutic options [54, 55].

Turmeric is composed of plant compounds that possess antioxidant, anti-inflammatory, and antimicrobial activities. Curcumin can lower inflammatory markers such TNF (tumor necrosis factor) and IL-6 (interleukin-6). Curcumin downregulates inflammatory pathways, including cyclooxygenase-2 (COX-2) and lipoxygenase, and inhibits transcription factor NF-kB, decreasing TNF-alfa and interleukin-1 (IL-1). Via these mechanisms, curcumin has broad antioxidant activity because it has a dual action: as a scavenger of free radicals and as a booster of endogenous antioxidant levels like glutathione and hemoxygenase-1, therefore improving cellular defenses against oxidative stress [56]. Curcumin was also shown to be an anti-androgen, an interesting property that can play a role in acne treatment.

Although its biologic activity is recognized, it has poor bioavailability. Studies have demonstrated that coadministration of curcumin and piperine, a substance found in black pepper, can increase plasma levels by upregulating bioavailability [56]. Turmeric can be recommended as an adjuvant for painful and inflammatory rosacea symptoms.

References

1. Zamani M, Neghab N, Torabian S. Therapeutic effect of Vitex agnus-castus in patients with premenstrual syndrome. Acta Med Iran. 2012;50(2):101–6.
2. Norman RA. Integrative dermatology. Oxford: Oxford University Press; 2014.
3. Nasri H, Bahmani M, Shahinfard N, Moradi Nafchi A, Saberianpour S, Rafieian KM. Medicinal plants for the treatment of acne vulgaris: a review of recent evidences. Jundishapur J Microbiol. 2015;8(11):e25580.
4. Wu Y, Li RW, Huang H, Fletcher A, Yu L, Pham Q, et al. Inhibition of tumor growth by dietary indole-3-carbinol in a prostate cancer xenograft model may be associated with disrupted gut microbial interactions. Nutrients. 2019;11(2):467.
5. Licznerska B, Baer-Dubowska W. Indole-3-carbinol and its role in chronic diseases. In: Gupta SC, Prasad S, Aggarwal BB, editors. Anti-inflammatory nutraceuticals and chronic diseases. Philadelphia: Springer; 2016. p. 131–54.
6. Katz E, Nisani S, Chamovitz DA. Indole-3-carbinol: a plant hormone combatting cancer. F1000Res. 2018;7. https://doi.org/10.12688/f1000research.14127.1.
7. Schulz V, Hänsel R, Blumenthal M, Tyler VE. Rational phytotherapy: a reference guide for physicians and pharmacists. Heidelberg: Springer; 2004.
8. Christie S, Walker AF. Vitex agnus-castus L. A review of its traditional and modern therapeutic use, current use from a survey of practitioners. Eur J Herb Med. 1997;3:29–45.
9. Du Mee C. Vitex agnus castus. Aust J Med Herbalism. 1993;5(3):63–5.
10. Blumenthal MJ. The complete German commission E monographs. Integrative Medicine Communication, 1999.
11. Kuruüzüm-Uz A, Ströch K, Demirezer LÖ, Zeeck A. Glucosides from Vitex agnus-castus. Phytochemistry. 2003;63(8):959–64.
12. Newall CA, Anderson LA, Phillipson JD. Herbal medicines. A guide for health-care professionals. London: Pharmaceutical Press; 1996.
13. Boon H, Smith M. The botanical pharmacy: the pharmacology of 47 common herbs. Kingston: Quarry press; 1999.
14. Sliutz G, Speiser P, Schultz AM, Spona J, Zeillinger R. Agnus castus extracts inhibit prolactin secretion of rat pituitary cells. Horm Metab Res. 1993;25(5):253–5.

15. Jarry H, Leonhardt S, Gorkow C, Wuttke WJ. In vitro prolactin but not LH and FSH release is inhibited by compounds in extracts of Agnus castus: direct evidence for a dopaminergic principle by the dopamine receptor assay. Exp Clin Endocrinol. 1994;102(6):448–54.
16. Wuttke W, Gorkow C, Jarry H. Dopaminergic compounds in Vitex agnus castus. In: Loew D, Rietbrock N, editors. Phytopharmaka in Forschung und klinischer Anwendung. Heidelberg: Steinkopff; 1995. p. 81–91.
17. Serri O, Chik CL, Ur E, Ezzat SJC. Diagnosis and management of hyperprolactinemia. CMAJ. 2003;169(6):575–81.
18. Daniele C, Coon JT, Pittler MH, Ernst EJ. Vitex agnus castus: a systematic review of adverse events. Drug Saf. 2005;28(4):319–32.
19. Loch EG, Selle H, Boblitz N. Treatment of premenstrual syndrome with a phytopharmaceutical formulation containing Vitex agnus castus. J Womens Health Gend Based Med. 2000;9(3):315–20.
20. Berger D, Schaffner W, Schrader E, Meier B, Brattstrom A. Efficacy of Vitex agnus castus L. extract Ze 440 in patients with pre-menstrual syndrome (PMS). Arch Gynecol Obstet. 2000;264(3):150–3.
21. van Die MD, Burger HG, Teede HJ, Bone KM. Vitex agnus-castus (Chaste-Tree/Berry) in the treatment of menopause-related complaints. J Altern Complement Med. 2009;15(8):853–62.
22. Atmaca M, Kumru S, Tezcan E. Fluoxetine versus Vitex agnus castus extract in the treatment of premenstrual dysphoric disorder. Hum Psychopharmacol. 2003;18(3):191–5.
23. Freeman EW. Premenstrual syndrome and premenstrual dysphoric disorder: definitions and diagnosis. Psychoneuroendocrinology. 2003;28(Suppl 3):25–37.
24. Lauritzen C, Reuter HD, Repges R, Bohnert KJ, Schmidt U. Treatment of premenstrual tension syndrome with Vitex agnus castus controlled, double-blind study versus pyridoxine. Phytomedicine. 1997;4(3):183–9.
25. Bedi MK, Shenefelt PD. Herbal therapy in dermatology. Arch Dermatol. 2002;138(2):232–42.
26. Tarkowská D, Strnad M. Plant ecdysteroids; plant sterols with intriguing distributions biological effects and relations to plant hormones. Planta. 2016;244(3):545–55.
27. Kaur P, Robin, Makanjuola VO, Arora R, Singh B, Arora S. Immunopotentiating significance of conventionally used plants adaptogens as modulators in biochemical and molecu-

lar signaling pathways in cell mediated processes. Biomed Pharmacother. 2017;95:1815–29.
28. Chen Y, Lyga J. Brain-skin connection: stress, inflammation and skin aging. Inflamm Allergy Drug Targets. 2014;13(3):177–90.
29. Bhuchar S, Katta R, Wolf J. Complementary and alternative medicine in dermatology: an overview of selected modalities for the practicing dermatologist. Am J Clin Dermatol. 2012;13(5):311–7.
30. Dobrek T. The outline of stress pathophysiology and pharmacodynamic action of plant based eustressors - adaptogens. Pol Merkur Lekarski. 2019;46(273):103–8.
31. National Rosacea Society. Studies find rosacea may lead to increased oxidative stress, 2019. Available at: http://www.rosacea.org/blog/2019/april/study-finds-rosacea-may-lead-increased-oxidative-stress-041519.
32. Sener S, Akbas A, Kilinc F, Baran P, Erel O, Aktas A. Thiol/disulfide homeostasis as a marker of oxidative stress in rosacea: a controlled spectrophotometric study. Cutan Ocul Toxicol. 2019;38(1):55–8.
33. Gur TF, Erdemir AV, Gurel MS, Kocyigit A, Guler EM, Erdil D. The investigation of the relationships of Demodex density with inflammatory response and oxidative stress in rosacea. Arch Dermatol Res. 2018;310(9):759–67.
34. Zoubolis CC, Seltmann H, Hiroi N, Chen WC, Young M, Oeff M, et al. Corticotropin-releasing hormone: an autocrine hormone that promotes lipogenesis in human sebocytes. Proc Natl Acad Sci U S A. 2002;99(10):7148–53.
35. Zhou CL, Yu X-J, Chen L-M, Jiang H, Li C-Y. Corticotropin-releasing hormone attenuates vascular endothelial growth factor release from human HaCaT keratinocytes. Regul Pept. 2010;160(1–3):115–20.
36. Zhong X, Lin S, Funk WE, Hou L. Environmental occupational exposure to chemicals and telomere length in human studies. Occup Environ Med. 2013;70(10):743–9.
37. Boesten DM, de Vos-Houben JM, Timmermans L, den Hartog GJM, Bast A, Hageman GJ. Accelerated aging during chronic oxidative stress: a role for PARP-1. Oxidative Med Cell Longev. 2013;2013:680414. https://doi.org/10.1155/2013/680414.
38. Tyrka AR, Price LH, Kao H-T, Porton B, Marsella SA, Carpenter LL. Childhood maltreatment and telomere shortening: preliminary support for an effect of early stress on cellular aging. Biol Psychiatry. 2010;67(6):531–4.

39. Panossian A. Understanding adaptogenic activity: specificity of the pharmacological action of adaptogens and other phytochemicals. Ann N Y Acad Sci. 2017;1401(1):49–64.
40. Panossian A, Wickman G, Sarris J. Rosenroot (Rhodiola rosea): traditional use, chemical composition, pharmacology and clinical efficacy. Phytomedicine. 2010;17(7):481–93.
41. Kosakowska O, Bączek K, Przybył JL, Pióro-Jabrucka E, Czupa W, Synowiec A, et al. Antioxidant and antibacterial activity of Rose root (Rhodiola rosea L.) dry extracts. Molecules. 2018;23(7):1767.
42. Zhou Q, Yin Z-P, Ma L, Zhao W, Hao H-W, Li H-L. Free radical-scavenging activities of oligomeric proanthocyanidin from Rhodiola rosea L. and its antioxidant effects in vivo. Nat Prod Res. 2014;28(24):1–3.
43. Committee on Herbal Medicinal Products. Community herbal monograph on Rhodiola rosea L., Rhizoma ex Radix. Committee on herbal medicine. London: European Medicines Agency; 2012.
44. Committee on Herbal Medicinal Products. Reflection paper on the adaptogenic concept. London: European Medicines Agency; 2008.
45. Ma Y-C, Wang X-Q, Hou FF, Ma J, Luo M, Lu S, et al. Rapid resolution liquid chromatography (RRLC) analysis for quality control of Rhodiola rosea roots and commercial standardized products. Nat Prod Commun. 2011;6(5):645–50.
46. Kim J. Review of the innate immune response in acne vulgaris: activation of toll -like receptor2 in acne triggers inflammatory cytokine responses. Dermatology (Basel). 2005;211:193–8.
47. Abeyama K, Eng W, Jester JV, Vink AA, Edelbaum D, Cockerell CJ, et al. A role for NF-Kappa B- dependent gene transactivation in sunburn. J Clin Invest. 2000;105(12):1751–9.
48. Guo M, An F, Wei X, Hong M, Lu Y. Comparative effects of schisandrin A,B and C on acne related inflammation. Inflammation. 2017;40(6):2063–172.
49. Lam PY, Yan CW, Chiu PY, Leung HY, Ko KM. Schisandrin B protects against solar irradiation-induced oxidative stress in rat skin tissue. Fitoterapia. 2011;82(3):393–400.
50. Guo M, Lu Y, Yang J, Zhao X, Lu Y. Inhibitory effects of Schisandra chinensis extract on acne-related inflammation and UVB-induced photo-aging. Pharm Biol. 2016;54(12):2987–94.
51. Bhattacharya SK, Kaur R, Ghosal S. Antistress activity of sitoindosides VII and VIII: new acylsterylglusides from Withania somnifera. Phytother Res. 1987;1:32–7.

52. Oláh A, Markovics A, Szabó-Papp J, Szabó PT, Stott C, Zoubouliset CC, et al. Differential effectiveness of selected non -psychotropic phytocannabinoids on human sebocyte functions implicates their introduction in dry/seborrheic skin and acne treatment. Exp Dermatol. 2016;25(9):701–7.
53. Oláh A, Rolf P, Biró T. Cannabidiol exerts sebostatic and anti-inflammatory effects on human sebocytes. J Clin Invest. 2014;124(9):3713–24.
54. Sishodia S. Molecular mechanisms of curcumin action: gene expression. Biofactors. 2013;39(1):37–55.
55. Nakamura K, Yasunaga Y, Segawa T, Ko D, Moul JW, Srivastava S, et al. Curcumin down-regulates AR gene expression and activation in prostate cell lines. Int J Oncol. 2002;21(4):825–30.
56. Shoba G, Joy D, Joseph T, Majeed M, Rajendran R, Srinivas PS. Influence of piperine on the pharmacokinetics of curcumin in animals and human volunteers. Planta Med. 1998;64(4):353–6.

Chapter 4
Topical Botanicals in Acne and Rosacea

Joanna N. Hooten and Lauren Schwartzberg

Green Tea

Green tea is a popular botanical across the world (Fig. 4.1). It accounts for about 20% of total tea production and is the end product of steaming and drying fresh leaves of the tea plant, *Camellia sinensis*, without damaging the polyphenolic compounds by oxidation or polymerization. Research on the health benefits of green tea has focused largely on systemic or topical administration of the phenolic fraction of green tea (GTP). The polyphenolic components of green tea include flavanols—also known as catechins—flavonoids, and phenolic acids, with flavanols existing in the highest concentration. The four major flavanols/catechins in green tea are (−)-epicatechin (EC), (−)-epicatechin-3-gallate (ECG), (−)-epigallocatechin (EG), and (−)-epigallocatechin-3-gallate (EGCG), which is the most active form [1]. GTPs have a broad range of clinical application in treating disease and senescence.

Oxidative stress is a major contributor to skin aging and disease, including malignancy [1]. The polyphenolic structure

J. N. Hooten (✉)
Clara Dermatology, Cary, NC, USA

L. Schwartzberg
New York Institute of Technology College of Osteopathic Medicine, Old Westbury, NY, USA

R. N. Rupani, P. A. Lio (eds.), *Integrative Dermatology*,
https://doi.org/10.1007/978-3-030-58954-7_4

FIGURE 4.1
Green Tea

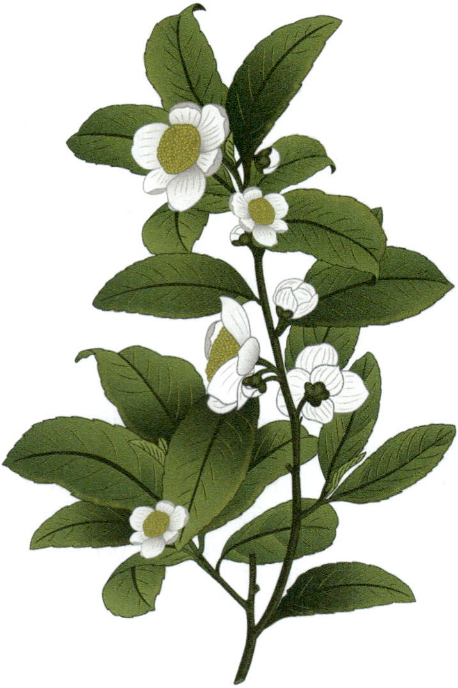

of GTPs enables them to scavenge free radicals and in humans and animals has been shown to reduce markers of oxidative stress including lipid peroxidation and protein carbonylation [2, 3]. Oxidative stress can lead to activation of mitogen-activated protein kinases (MAPK), triggering proinflammatory cytokine pathways [4]. Anti-inflammatory properties of GTPs have been linked to the MAPK pathway and downstream activity of matrix metalloproteinases, growth factor activity, and DNA stability [4–8]. GTPs, even topically applied, can also inhibit growth factor signaling and unregulated DNA turnover, impacting key aspects in cell cycle and turnover [9–12]. These properties have led to research and clinical application of GTPs in a variety of skin disorders. Although much of the current literature is based on in vitro or systemic administration of GTPs, several studies have been done on beneficial effects of topical application in acne and rosacea, which is the focus of this volume.

Acne affects over 50 million Americans per year, making it the most common skin condition in the United States [13]. Acne is a chronic, multifactorial process involving excessive sebaceous gland activity and hormonal stimulation, altered keratinization of the hair follicles, bacterial overgrowth due to proliferation of *Cutibacterium acnes (formerly Propionibacterium acnes*), and inflammation [14]. The pro-inflammatory effects of *C. acnes* are mediated through the toll-like receptor 2 (TLR2) and subsequent release of pro-inflammatory cytokines [15]. Polyphenon-60, a GTP, was shown to suppress TLR2 expression and IL-8 secretion [16]. In vitro and in vivo topical applications of EGCG have been shown to decrease sebaceous gland size, suppress sebocyte proliferation and lipogenesis, and suppress IL-1, IL-6, and IL-8 [17]. Green tea extract has been shown to have antimicrobial effects on *C. acnes*, *Staphylococcus aureus*, and *Staphylococcus epidermidis* [18]. In a split-face trial of 22 participants, an emulsion containing 5% green tea extract, applied topically for 60 days, significantly decreased sebum secretion compared with placebo [19]. Another study found that EGCG reduced sebum production, induced sebocyte apoptosis, and decreased *C. acnes*-induced inflammation. The same study enrolled 35 acne patients in an 8-week split-face trial of topical application of 1% or 5% EGCG solution vs. vehicle and found that topical treatment of EGCG was well tolerated and significantly decreased inflammatory and non-inflammatory acne lesions [20]. Similarly, topical application of lotion containing 2% green tea lead to statistically significant improvement in papulopustular acne after twice-daily application for 2 months [21].

Rosacea is a chronic inflammatory skin disorder resulting in hypersensitive skin due to dysregulation of the innate immune system by various factors, including prostaglandins and reactive oxygen species (ROS) [22]. Erythema and telangiectasia, key clinical features of rosacea, can be an end result of aberrant stimulation of vascular endothelial growth factor (VEGF) via hypoxia-inducible factor-1 (HIF-1). EGCG has been shown to decrease VEGF and HIF-1 expression in vitro [23]. A 6-week trial of 2.5% EGCG cream applied twice daily on subjects with facial erythema and telangiectasia resulted in significant reduction of VEGF and HIF-1. Although no clinical improvement in erythema was found in this short study, this may be an evolving topic for research.

Turmeric

Turmeric is a spice derived from the ground roots of *Curcuma longa*, a plant grown chiefly in Asia and Central America (Fig. 4.2). The main biologically active ingredient in turmeric is curcumin, a phytopolylphenol pigment that gives turmeric its yellow color. Curcumin accounts for 3–4% of turmeric by weight [24]. Turmeric and its components have

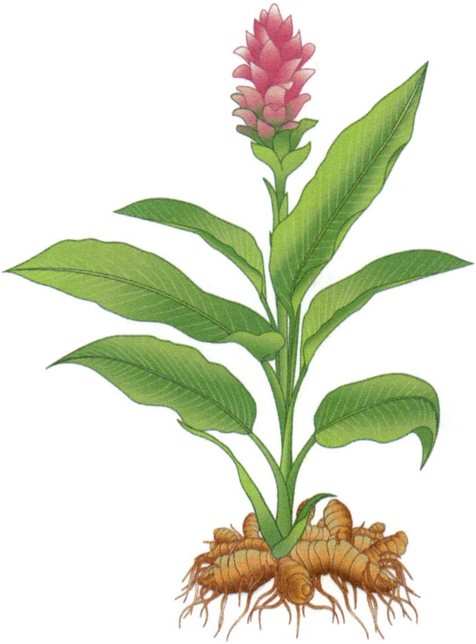

FIGURE 4.2
Turmeric

anti-inflammatory, antimicrobial, antioxidant, and antineoplastic properties and have been used in Asia for a variety of skin disorders [25, 26]. The use of curcumin for inflammatory skin conditions, including acne and rosacea, is often part of a complementary or alternative medicine approach [27].

Many of the anti-inflammatory effects of curcumin have been studied in the rheumatoid arthritis model, which shares many of the same mediators as acne and rosacea. These include TNFα, nuclear factor kappa B (NFkB), cytokines, and prostaglandins [28, 29]. Topically applying biodegradable microspheres of curcumin improved inflammatory arthritis in rats and significantly decreased swelling in the carrageenan-induced rat paw edema, which serves as the standard model for studying acute inflammation [30–33]. Additionally, patients treated with curcumin had clinical improvement in arthritis [34]. More specifically, curcumin has been shown to decrease TNFα and NFkB activation; the oxidative metabolites of curcumin accounted for the bulk of activity against NFkB [35]. Curcumin also decreases IL-8, via moderation of TLR2 [36, 37]. The enzymatic activity of cyclooxygenase 2 (COX-2) was also suppressed by curcumin, leading to diminished production of prostaglandins, which promote inflammation in rosacea [38, 39]. Curcumin inhibits formation ROS, which cause cell damage in many processes including acne and rosacea [40–42]. Beyond antioxidant properties, in vitro studies have shown high concentrations of curcumin were effective against various pathogenic bacteria including *S. aureus*, *S. epidermidis*, *Pseudomonas aeruginosa*, *Escherichia coli*, *Enterococcus faecalis*, and *Bacillus subtilis* [43, 44]. Curcumin has also been shown to inhibit the growth of *C. acnes* [45]. Furthermore, the combination of blue light therapy and topical curcumin was found to be cytotoxic to *C. acnes* [46]. A study comparing turmeric and lauric acid in a liposomal gel formulation with azithromycin found that the combination of turmeric and lauric acid had enhanced antibacterial activity against macrolide sensitive and resistant strains of *C. acnes* and reduced cytokine production and comedones when applied topically to rat ear skin [47].

In humans, a study of 153 patients found that treatment with an oral tablet containing neem, curcumin, and piper extract and a tea tree oil gel was significantly more helpful in treating acne than either treatment alone [48]. Another study, using a polyherbal gel facial wash containing curcumin and neem, found it to be nearly as effective as clindamycin gel in acne patients [49, 50]. Additionally, a study of 13 patients using a topical cream containing 5% turmeric or control applied twice daily to facial skin for 12 weeks found significantly reduced sebum production in areas treated with turmeric [51]. These findings suggest turmeric may be effective against various mechanisms involved in acne, making it a promising adjunctive therapy.

Curcumin is well tolerated in animals and humans. Suprapharmacological doses of curcumin essential oil complex (5000 mg/kg/day) showed no acute toxicity in animals, and high doses of the same preparation (1000 mg/kg/day) did not show significant side effects [52]. A clinical trial of curcumin in humans showed no significant toxicity [53].

Chamomile

Matricaria chamomilla, commonly known as chamomile, is a daisy-like plant in the *Asteraceae* family with two main species of pharmacological interest (Fig. 4.3). *Matricaria chamomilla* (syn. *Matricaria recutita*), also known as German chamomile, is better studied than the Roman chamomile variety, also known as *Chamaemelum nobile*. Chamomile has been called "physician of plants" and its medicinal use dates back to Hippocrates and Galen [54]. The growing interest in chamomile has fueled research on its antimicrobial, anti-inflammatory, and antioxidant properties.

Over 120 components have been identified in its oil, the most significant are terpenoids, bisabolol, chamazulene, β-farnesene, and α bisabolol oxides A and B; flavonoids, apigenin, quercetin, patuletin, and luteolin; and sesquiterpenes, coumarin, tannins, polysaccharides, choline, and phytoestrogens [55].

FIGURE 4.3
Chamomile

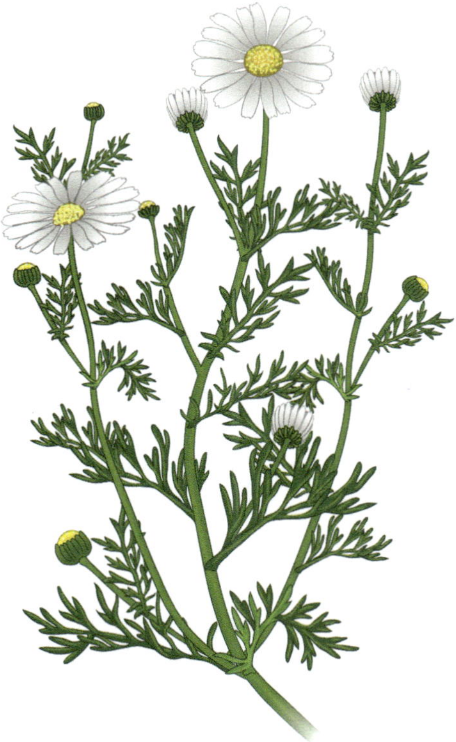

The effectual essence of this plant is a blue oil derived from the sesquiterpenes in its flowers, but the chemical composition and medicinal efficacy of chamomile varies by species, type of soil, timing of cultivation, amount of sunlight and irrigation, and the presence of nitrogen. For example, chamomile in teabags, flowers, and purchases from a pharmacy shows a substantial difference in the chemical components and their percentages. Sesquiterpene hydrocarbons made up 58% of the pharmacy sample, whereas it was only 5–12% of the teabags and flowers. Teabags and flowers had nearly three times as much chamazulene and bisabolol compounds as the pharmacy product [56]. As with many herbal preparations, effectiveness relies on accurate formulations of active compounds isolated from chamomile [55].

Important sesquiterpenes isolated from chamomile include farnesol, bisabolol, and chamazulene. These are lipophilic compounds that have numerous biological effects, including anti-inflammatory, analgesic, and neuroprotective. There is also interest in their potential effectiveness as absorption enhancers, as co-administering these compounds with topical antibiotics may facilitate absorption [57, 58]. Interestingly, chamomile oil increased the dermal absorption of caffeine by threefold and acetylsalicylic acid by twofold [59].

A combination of *M. chamomilla*, *J. regia*, *M. communis*, *Urtica dioica* (nettle leaves), and *Rosa damascena* (rose flowers) was tested on a both a pharmaceutically supplied isolate of *P. acnes* and a clinical isolate. Strong antibacterial reactions were evident by the minimum inhibitory concentration (MIC) of 0.048%v/v scores for both tests [60]. However, several other studies of *M. chamomilla* alone have not found it to be effective against *C. acnes*, *S. aureus*, or *S. epidermidis* [61–64].

Chamomile shows good antioxidant properties compared to ascorbic acid [61]. Free radical scavenging and β-*carotene*–linoleic acid assays showed the essential oil chamomile has significant antioxidant activity [65]. Another study showed that a significant amount of the antioxidant activity of chamomile can be attributed to chamazulene [66]. Additionally, bisabolol has been shown to inhibit free radical formation in human skin fibroblasts [67]. An aqueous extract of chamomile led to inhibition of COX-2 gene expression as well as direct blockage of COX-2 enzymatic activity, decreasing prostaglandin production [68]. The less commonly studied species of chamomile, *C. nobile*, containing predominantly α-bisabolol and farnesene, was found to have anti-inflammatory activity similar to that of ibuprofen [69]. α-Bisabolol was shown to inhibit TNFα and IL-6 and clinically reduce skin edema in mice [70]. Based on a review of in vivo skin studies, German chamomile (GC) oil demonstrates a definitive anti-inflammatory effect and a possible effect on skin barrier repair [71].

These studies suggest chamomile has potent antioxidant and anti-inflammatory properties, which may facilitate management of acne and rosacea.

Neem

Azadirachta indica is the scientific name for the neem tree, which is native to the Indian subcontinent and has been used for medicinal purposes for millennia (Fig. 4.4). Siddha medicine is one of the oldest healthcare systems in the world, dating

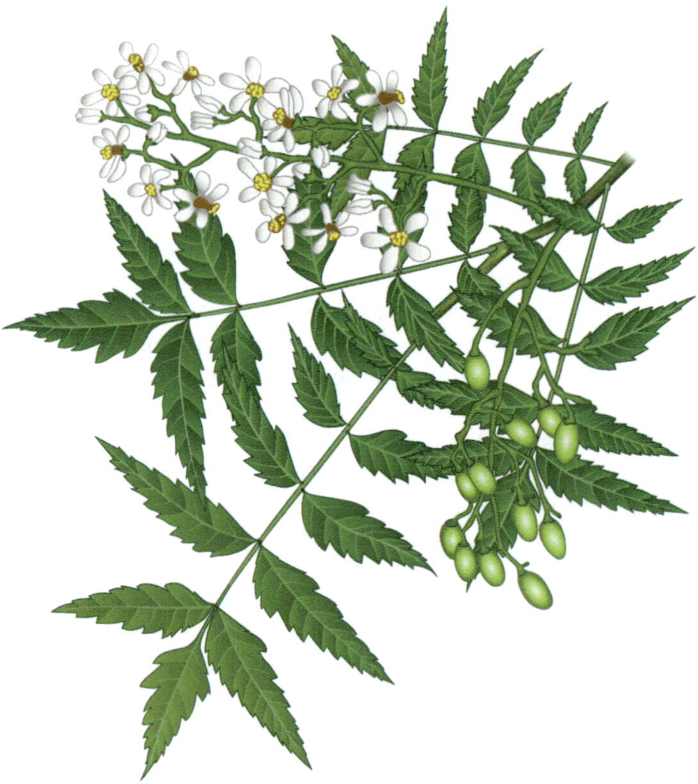

FIGURE 4.4 Neem

between 10,000 and 4000 B.C., and one of the earliest medicinal plants mentioned in this ancient medical system is neem [72]. Neem extract and oil have been used both orally and topically as treatment for numerous ailments including periodontal disease, skin disorders, diabetes, ulcers, inflammatory conditions, and infections [73, 74]. Neem is a rich source of limonoids, which have potent antioxidant, anti-inflammatory, and antineoplastic properties [75]. The biologically active compounds within neem include azadirachtin, nimbin, nimbidin, nimbolides, mahmoodin, and cyclic trisulfide [76].

Neem has been shown to inhibit the various inflammatory mediators of acne and rosacea. Neem extract reduced inflammation via NFkB, which subsequently decreased TNFα activity [77]. As discussed previously, TNFα, TLR2, and cytokines are key mediators of inflammation in acne [78]. Neem leaf extract significantly reduced the serotonin and prostaglandin-mediated inflammation in the carrageenan-induced rat hind paw edema model; both mediate inflammation in rosacea [79]. Neem seed oil exhibited a dose-dependent inhibition of carrageenan-induced rat hind paw edema, with maximal effect at the third to fourth hour [80]. This pharmacokinetic profile is very similar to that of acetylsalicylic acid, which blocks prostaglandin production via the COX pathway. Additionally, nimbidin, one of the active ingredients in neem, suppressed macrophage and neutrophil activity, both key players in the inflammatory process in acne and rosacea [81, 82].

Neem has exhibited in vitro activity against *S. aureus* and other bacteria, but did not significantly inhibit *C. acnes*, the main pathogenic bacteria in acne [83, 84]. However, the inflammatory mediators of infection with *C. acnes* are inhibited by neem in vitro [85]. This discrepancy between the inability to directly inhibit *C. acnes* infection and the ability to suppress inflammatory mediators of *C. acnes* supports the theory that the effectiveness of antibiotic treatment of skin disorders may have more to do with the anti-inflammatory activity than the antimicrobial activity [86].

A clinical study of 29 patients demonstrated efficacy only in some stages of acne after 6 months of treatment with an oral preparation of *A. indica*. Although there was a significant reduction in the overall number of lesions, improvement in the Global Acne Grading System score, and improvement in the Acne-specific Quality of Life questionnaire, it did not reduce the number of inflammatory lesions of acne. The study concluded that *A. indica* was effective for the early and recovery stages of acne, but not the inflammatory stage [87].

A toxicity study of parenterally applied neem oil in rats and rabbits showed no adverse events at doses of 177 and 537 mg/kg per day for 90 days. However, there were significant side effects in the liver, kidneys, and testes at doses of 1600 mg/kg per day [88].

Viburnum

Viburnum is a genus of over 150 species of flowering plants in the family *Adoxaceae*, whose member species are evergreen or deciduous shrubs that are common in temperate climates in the Northern Hemisphere and some areas of South America, Asia, and Africa, particularly *Viburnum opulus* (Fig. 4.5) [89]. The shrubs are most commonly used as ornamental plants and have a fruit that is a flesh berry. They also may also be referred to as cranberry bush fruit or gilaburu. Polyphenols have been isolated from many viburnum species, mainly from the fruit skin, but the phenolic content depends on environmental conditions [90–93].

V. opulus, also known as cramp bark, is common in North American and Europe and contains proanthocyanidins and viopudial, which has antispasmodic effects on smooth muscle [94]. *V. mullaha*, which is found in Indian Himalayan region, has anti-elastase and anti-collagenase activities, and anti-tyrosinase activity. *V. mullaha* was also found to contain 15 phenolic compounds and 13 flavonoids, including chlorogenic acid, dihydromyricetin, rutin, dihydroquercetin, theaflavin, and epicatechin [95]. *V. opulus* contains phenolic compounds, the highest in concentration being coumaroylquinic acid, chlorogenic acid, procyanidin B2, and procyanidin trimer

FIGURE 4.5
Viburnum

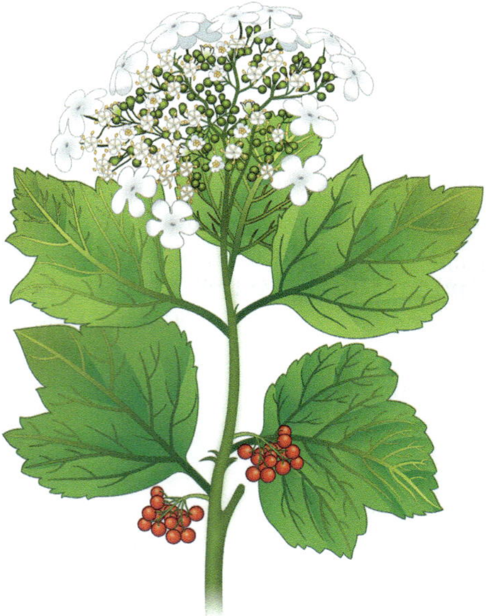

[90]. Given the abundance of polyphenols in viburnum plants, topical formulations are likely to be beneficial to many skin processes, particularly processes that involve oxidative damage and hyperpigmentation, such as acne. Viburnum extract is a component in many cosmeceuticals skin products, but evidence-based research on the effect of topical application needs further exploration.

Nettles

Urtica dicoa, often referred to as nettle, is an herbaceous diclinous plant from the *Urticaceae* family that is commonly found in warm, tropical regions (Fig. 4.6) [96]. Although known in dermatology as a cause of contact urticaria, extracts from nettles have been shown to have antioxidant and antimicrobial properties [97]. Nettle extracts have been used

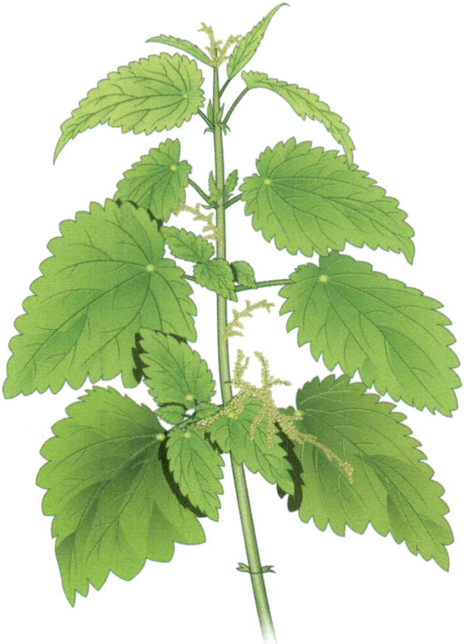

FIGURE 4.6
Nettle

for medicinal purposes in benign prostatic hypertrophy via hormonal modulation, bladder infections, and as an effective alternative to nonsteroidal anti-inflammatory drugs [98–100]. Nettle has been found to be helpful in inflammatory arthritis through moderation of the cytokine profile, and allergic rhinitis, by inhibition of cyclooxygenases and prostaglandins [101, 102]. Phenolic compounds isolated from nettle may also protect against diabetes [103]. As mentioned previously, a combination extract containing walnut husk, myrtle leaves, chamomilla flower, and nettle leaves was to be effective against *C. acnes* and suppressed activity of TNFα in human keratinocytes in vitro [60]. Similar to viburnum, more definitive studies are needed. Many properties of nettle suggest it has the ability to target pathogenic mechanisms in acne and rosacea.

Conclusion

Plant-derived compounds have powerful effects on inflammation and can protect against bacterial activity, excessive sebum production, and the sequelae of inflammation. Although green tea and turmeric have the greatest level of evidence, components of chamomile, neem, viburnum, and nettle also have properties that may prove beneficial as part of a successful integrative approach to treating acne and rosacea.

References

1. Katiyar SK, Mukhtar H. Tea antioxidants in cancer chemoprevention. J Cell Biochem. 1997;67(S27):59–67.
2. Valcic S, Burr JA, Timmermann BN, Liebler DC. Antioxidant chemistry of green tea catechins. New oxidation products of (−)-epigallocatechin gallate and (−)-epigallocatechin from their reactions with peroxyl radicals. Chem Res Toxicol. 2000;13(9):801–10.
3. Senthil Kumaran V, Arulmathi K, Srividhya R, Kalaiselvi P. Repletion of antioxidant status by EGCG and retardation of oxidative damage induced macromolecular anomalies in aged rats. Exp Gerontol. 2008;43(3):176–83.
4. Ondet T, Muscatelli-Groux B, Coulouarn C, Robert S, Gicquel T, Bodin A, et al. The release of pro-inflammatory cytokines is mediated via mitogen-activated protein kinases rather than by the inflammasome signalling pathway in keratinocytes. Clin Exp Pharmacol Physiol. 2017;44(7):827–38.
5. Kim HS, Kim MH, Jeong M, Hwang YS, Lim SH, Shin BA, et al. EGCG blocks tumor promoter-induced MMP-9 expression via suppression of MAPK and AP-1 activation in human gastric AGS cells. Anticancer Res. 2004;24(2B):747–53.
6. Abd El-Rahman SS, Shehab G, Nashaat H. Epigallocatechin-3-gallate: the prospective targeting of cancer stem cells and preventing metastasis of chemically-induced mammary cancer in rats. Am J Med Sci. 2017;354(1):54–63.
7. Li Y-F, Wang H, Fan Y, Shi H-J, Wang Q-M, Chen B-R, et al. Epigallocatechin-3-gallate inhibits matrix metalloproteinase-9

and monocyte chemotactic protein-1 expression through the 67-κDa laminin receptor and the TLR4/MAPK/NF-κB signalling pathway in lipopolysaccharide-induced macrophages. Cell Physiol Biochem. 2017;43(3):926–36.

8. Bae J-Y, Choi J-S, Choi Y-J, Shin S-Y, Kang S-W, Han SJ, et al. (−)Epigallocatechin gallate hampers collagen destruction and collagenase activation in ultraviolet-B-irradiated human dermal fibroblasts: involvement of mitogen-activated protein kinase. Food Chem Toxicol. 2008;46(4):1298–307.
9. Byun E-B, Choi H-G, Sung N-Y, Byun E-H. Green tea polyphenol epigallocatechin-3-gallate inhibits TLR4 signaling through the 67-kDa laminin receptor on lipopolysaccharide-stimulated dendritic cells. Biochem Biophys Res Commun. 2012;426(4):480–5.
10. Hong Byun E, Fujimura Y, Yamada K, Tachibana H. TLR4 signaling inhibitory pathway induced by green tea polyphenol epigallocatechin-3-gallate through 67-kDa laminin receptor. J Immunol. 2010;185(1):33–45.
11. Katiyar SK, Agarwal R, Mukhtar H. Protection against malignant conversion of chemically induced benign skin papillomas to squamous cell carcinomas in SENCAR mice by a polyphenolic fraction isolated from green tea. Cancer Res. 1993;53(22):5409–12.
12. Kumazoe M, Yamashita M, Nakamura Y, Takamatsu K, Bae J, Yamashita S, et al. Green tea polyphenol EGCG upregulates tollip expression by suppressing Elf-1 expression. J Immunol. 2017;199(9):3261–9.
13. Bickers DR, Lim HW, Margolis D, Weinstock MA, Goodman C, Faulkner E, et al. The burden of skin diseases: 2004 a joint project of the American Academy of Dermatology Association and the Society for Investigative Dermatology. J Am Acad Dermatol. 2006;55(3):490–500.
14. Cong T-X, Hao D, Wen X, Li X-H, He G, Jiang X. From pathogenesis of acne vulgaris to anti-acne agents. Arch Dermatol Res [Internet]. 2019 Mar 11. Available from: https://doi.org/10.1007/s00403-019-01908-x. [cited 2019 Apr 8].
15. Jugeau S, Tenaud I, Knol AC, Jarrousse V, Quereux G, Khammari A, et al. Induction of toll-like receptors by Propionibacterium acnes. Br J Dermatol. 2005;153(6):1105–13.
16. Jung MK, Ha S, Son J-A, Song JH, Houh Y, Cho E, et al. Polyphenon-60 displays a therapeutic effect on acne by suppression of TLR2 and IL-8 expression via down-regulating the ERK1/2 pathway. Arch Dermatol Res. 2012;304(8):655–63.

17. Im M, Kim SY, Sohn KC, Choi DK, Lee Y, Seo YJ, et al. Epigallocatechin-3-gallate suppresses IGF-I-induced lipogenesis and cytokine expression in SZ95 sebocytes. J Invest Dermatol. 2012;132(12):2700–8.
18. Li Z, Summanen PH, Downes J, Corbett K, Komoriya T, Henning SM, et al. Antimicrobial activity of pomegranate and green tea extract on propionibacterium acnes, propionibacterium granulosum, staphylococcus aureus and staphylococcus epidermidis. J Drugs Dermatol. 2015;14(6):574–8.
19. Mahmood T, Akhtar N, Moldovan C. A comparison of the effects of topical green tea and lotus on facial sebum control in healthy humans. Hippokratia. 2013;17(1):64–7.
20. Yoon JY, Kwon HH, Min SU, Thiboutot DM, Suh DH. Epigallocatechin-3-gallate improves acne in humans by modulating intracellular molecular targets and inhibiting P. acnes. [Internet]. Available from: https://scholar.google.com/scholar_lookup?title=Epigallocatechin-3-gallate%20improves%20acne%20in%20humans%20by%20modulating%20intracellular%20molecular%20targets%20and%20inhibiting%20P.%20Acnes&author=Yoon,+J.Y.&author=Kwon,+H.H.&author=Min,+S.U.&author=Thiboutot,+D.M.&author=Suh,+D.H.&publication_year=2013&journal=J.+Investig.+Dermatol.&volume=133&pages=429%E2%80%93440&doi=10.1038/jid.2012.292&pmid=23096708. [cited 2019 Apr 8].
21. Sharquie KE, Noaimi AA, Al-Salih MM. Topical therapy of acne vulgaris using 2% tea lotion in comparison with 5% zinc sulphate solution. Saudi Med J. 2008;29(12):1757–61.
22. Two AM, Wu W, Gallo RL, Hata TR. Rosacea: part I. Introduction, categorization, histology, pathogenesis, and risk factors. J Am Acad Dermatol. 2015;72(5):749–58; quiz 759–60.
23. Zhang Q, Tang X, Lu Q, Zhang Z, Rao J, Le AD. Green tea extract and (−)-epigallocatechin-3-gallate inhibit hypoxia- and serum-induced HIF-1alpha protein accumulation and VEGF expression in human cervical carcinoma and hepatoma cells. Mol Cancer Ther. 2006;5(5):1227–38.
24. Chattopadhyay I, Biswas K, Bandyopadhyay U, Banerjee RK. Turmeric and curcumin: biological actions and medicinal applications. Curr Sci. 2004;87(1):10.
25. Vaughn AR, Branum A, Sivamani RK. Effects of turmeric (Curcuma longa) on skin health: a systematic review of the clinical evidence. Phytother Res. 2016;30(8):1243–64.

26. Gupta SC, Kismali G, Aggarwal BB. Curcumin, a component of turmeric: from farm to pharmacy. Biofactors. 2013;39(1):2–13.
27. Kallis PJ, Price A, Dosal JR, Nichols AJ, Keri J. A biologically based approach to acne and rosacea. J Drugs Dermatol. 2018;17(6):611–7.
28. Fattahi M, Mirshafiey A. Prostaglandins and rheumatoid arthritis. Arthritis. 2012;2012:239310.
29. McInnes IB, Schett G. The pathogenesis of rheumatoid arthritis. N Engl J Med. 2011;365(23):2205–19.
30. Winter CA, Risley EA, Nuss GW. Carrageenan-induced edema in hind paw of the rat as an assay for antiiflammatory drugs. Proc Soc Exp Biol Med. 1962;111:544–7.
31. Fehrenbacher JC, Vasko MR, Duarte DB. Models of inflammation: carrageenan- or complete Freund's Adjuvant (CFA)-induced edema and hypersensitivity in the rat. Curr Protoc Pharmacol. 2012;5:Unit5.4.
32. Kumar V, Lewis SA, Mutalik S, Shenoy DB, Venkatesh, Udupa N. Biodegradable microspheres of curcumin for treatment of inflammation. Indian J Physiol Pharmacol. 2002;46(2):209–17.
33. Rao TS, Basu N, Siddiqui HH. Anti-inflammatory activity of curcumin analogues. [Internet]. [cited 2019 Apr 22]. Available from: https://web.b.ebscohost.com/abstract?direct=true&profile=ehost&scope=site&authtype=crawler&jrnl=09715916&AN=91713388&h=GNduiZHIWPKlw6aI%2b7Z8%2f1yvBkwSWf6ijOCyTbkFckDEjyX%2fuyiGrbWg%2bmyFa7SQoilpIPa6Z3DVLZD08K4yog%3d%3d&crl=c&resultNs=AdminWebAuth&resultLocal=ErrCrlNotAuth&crlhashurl=login.aspx%3fdirect%3dtrue%26profile%3dehost%26scope%3dsite%26authtype%3dcrawler%26jrnl%3d09715916%26AN%3d91713388.
34. Chandran B, Goel A. A randomized, pilot study to assess the efficacy and safety of curcumin in patients with active rheumatoid arthritis. Phytother Res. 2012;26(11):1719–25.
35. Edwards RL, Luis PB, Varuzza PV, Joseph AI, Presley SH, Chaturvedi R, et al. The anti-inflammatory activity of curcumin is mediated by its oxidative metabolites. J Biol Chem. 2017;292(52):21243–52.
36. Chaudhary N, Ueno-Shuto K, Ono T, Ohira Y, Watanabe K, Nasu A, et al. Curcumin down-regulates toll-like receptor-2 gene expression and function in human cystic fibrosis bronchial epithelial cells. Biol Pharm Bull. 2019;42(3):489–95.
37. Hidaka H, Ishiko T, Furuhashi T, Kamohara H, Suzuki S, Miyazaki M, et al. Curcumin inhibits interleukin 8 production

and enhances interleukin 8 receptor expression on the cell surface. Cancer. 2002;95(6):1206–14.
38. Surh YJ, Chun KS, Cha HH, Han SS, Keum YS, Park KK, et al. Molecular mechanisms underlying chemopreventive activities of anti-inflammatory phytochemicals: down-regulation of COX-2 and iNOS through suppression of NF-kappa B activation. Mutat Res. 2001;480–481:243–68.
39. Goel A, Boland CR, Chauhan DP. Specific inhibition of cyclooxygenase-2 (COX-2) expression by dietary curcumin in HT-29 human colon cancer cells. Cancer Lett. 2001;172(2):111–8.
40. Ak T, Gülçin İ. Antioxidant and radical scavenging properties of curcumin. Chem Biol Interact. 2008;174(1):27–37.
41. Jones DA. Rosacea, reactive oxygen species, and azelaic acid. J Clin Aesthet Dermatol. 2009;2(1):26–30.
42. Mills OH, Criscito MC, Schlesinger TE, Verdicchio R, Szoke E. Addressing free radical oxidation in acne vulgaris. J Clin Aesthet Dermatol. 2016;9(1):25–30.
43. Gunes H, Gulen D, Mutlu R, Gumus A, Tas T, Topkaya AE. Antibacterial effects of curcumin: an in vitro minimum inhibitory concentration study. Toxicol Ind Health. 2016;32(2):246–50.
44. Hegge AB, Bruzell E, Kristensen S, Tønnesen HH. Photoinactivation of Staphylococcus epidermidis biofilms and suspensions by the hydrophobic photosensitizer curcumin--effect of selected nanocarrier: studies on curcumin and curcuminoides XLVII. Eur J Pharm Sci. 2012;47(1):65–74.
45. Liu C-H, Huang H-Y. In vitro anti-propionibacterium activity by curcumin containing vesicle system. Chem Pharm Bull. 2013;61(4):419–25.
46. Yang M-Y, Chang K-C, Chen L-Y, Hu A. Low-dose blue light irradiation enhances the antimicrobial activities of curcumin against Propionibacterium acnes. J Photochem Photobiol B. 2018;189:21–8.
47. Madan S, Nehate C, Barman TK, Rathore AS, Koul V. Design, preparation, and evaluation of liposomal gel formulations for treatment of acne: in vitro and in vivo studies. Drug Dev Ind Pharm. 2019;45(3):395–404.
48. Belemkar S. Evaluation of efficacy and safety of perfect face gel and perfect face tablets in management of acne. J Clin Exp Dermatol Res. 2011;10:2.
49. Rasheed A, Avinash Kumar Reddy G, Mohanalakshmi S, Ashok Kumar CK. Formulation and comparative evaluation of poly herbal anti-acne face wash gels. Pharm Biol. 2011;49(8):771–4.

50. Shaffrathul JH, Karthick PS, Rai R, Srinivas CR. Turmeric: role in hypertrichosis and acne. Indian J Dermatol. 2007;52(2):116.
51. Zaman SU, Akhtar N. Effect of turmeric (Curcuma longa Zingiberaceae) extract cream on human skin sebum secretion. Trop J Pharm Res. 2013;12(5):665–9.
52. Aggarwal ML, Chacko KM, Kuruvilla BT. Systematic and comprehensive investigation of the toxicity of curcuminoid-essential oil complex: a bioavailable turmeric formulation. Mol Med Rep. 2016;13(1):592–604.
53. Aggarwal BB, Kumar A, Bharti AC. Anticancer potential of curcumin: preclinical and clinical studies. Anticancer Res. 2003;23(1A):363–98.
54. Mohammad SM. Study on chamomile (Matricaria chamomilla L.) usage and farming. Adv Environ Biol. 2011;5:1446–53.
55. Singh O, Khanam Z, Misra N, Srivastava MK. Chamomile (Matricaria chamomilla L.): an overview. Pharmacogn Rev. 2011;5(9):82–95.
56. Farhoudi R. Chemical constituents and antioxidant properties of matricaria recutita and chamaemelum nobile essential oil growing wild in the south west of Iran. J Essent Oil Bear Plants. 2013;16(4):531–7.
57. Chadwick M, Trewin H, Gawthrop F, Wagstaff C. Sesquiterpenoids lactones: benefits to plants and people. Int J Mol Sci. 2013;14(6):12780–805. Available from: https://www.mdpi.com/1422-0067/14/6/12780/htm. [cited 2019 Apr 23].
58. Kamatou GPP, Viljoen AM. A review of the application and pharmacological properties of α-bisabolol and α-bisabolol-rich oils. J Am Oil Chem Soc. 2010;87(1):1–7.
59. Avonto C, Rua D, Lasonkar PB, Chittiboyina AG, Khan IA. Identification of a compound isolated from German chamomile (Matricaria chamomilla) with dermal sensitization potential. Toxicol Appl Pharmacol. 2017;318:16–22.
60. Kiliç S, Okullu SÖ, Kurt Ö, Sevinç H, Dündar C, Altınordu F, et al. Efficacy of two plant extracts against acne vulgaris: initial results of microbiological tests and cell culture studies. J Cosmet Dermatol. 2019;18(4):1061–5.
61. Vora J, Srivastava A, Modi H. Antibacterial and antioxidant strategies for acne treatment through plant extracts. Inform Med Unlocked. 2018;13:128–32.
62. Zu Y, Yu H, Liang L, Fu Y, Efferth T, Liu X, et al. Activities of ten essential oils towards Propionibacterium acnes and PC-3, A-549 and MCF-7 cancer cells. Molecules. 2010;15(5):3200–10.

63. Sakkas H, Economou V, Gousia P, Bozidis P, Sakkas VA, Petsios S, et al. Antibacterial efficacy of commercially available essential oils tested against drug-resistant gram-positive pathogens. Appl Sci. 2018;8(11):2201.
64. Soković M, Glamočlija J, Marin PD, Brkić D, van Griensven LJLD. Antibacterial effects of the essential oils of commonly consumed medicinal herbs using an in vitro model. Molecules. 2010;15(11):7532–46.
65. Abdoul-Latif F, Mohamed N, Edou P, Abdou Ali A, Djama SO, Obame Engonga L-C, et al. Antimicrobial and antioxidant activities of essential oil and methanol extract of Matricaria Chamomilla L. from Djibouti. J Med Plants Res. 2011;1:5.
66. Sizova NV. Composition and antioxidant activity of essential oils containing azulene derivatives. Pharm Chem J. 2012;46(6):369–71.
67. Mamalis A, Nguyen D-H, Brody N, Jagdeo J. The active natural anti-oxidant properties of chamomile, milk thistle, and halophilic bacterial components in human skin in vitro. J Drugs Dermatol. 2013;12(7):780–4.
68. Srivastava JK, Pandey M, Gupta S. Chamomile, a novel and selective COX-2 inhibitor with anti-inflammatory activity. Life Sci. 2009;85(19–20):663–9.
69. Aremu O, Tata C, Sewani-Rusike C, Oyedeji A, Oyedeji OO, Nkeh-Chungag B. Phytochemical composition, and analgesic and anti-inflammatory properties of essential oil of Chamaemelum nobile (Asteraceae L All) in rodents. Trop J Pharm Res. 2018;10:1939–45.
70. Maurya AK, Singh M, Dubey V, Srivastava S, Luqman S, Bawankule DU. α-(−)-bisabolol reduces pro-inflammatory cytokine production and ameliorates skin inflammation. Curr Pharm Biotechnol. 2014;15(2):173–81.
71. Lin T-K, Zhong L, Santiago JL. Anti-inflammatory and skin barrier repair effects of topical application of some plant oils. Int J Mol Sci. 2017;19(1):E70.
72. Kumar VS, Navaratnam V. Neem (Azadirachta indica): prehistory to contemporary medicinal uses to humankind. Asian Pac J Trop Biomed. 2013;3(7):505–14.
73. Tiwari R, Verma AK, Chakraborty S, Dhama K, Singh SV. Neem (Azadirachta indica) and its potential for safeguarding health of animals and humans: a review. [Internet]. Available from: https://scialert.net/abstract/?doi=jbs.2014.110.123. [cited 2019 Apr 22].
74. Prashant GM, Chandu GN, Murulikrishna KS, Shafiulla MD. The effect of mango and neem extract on four organisms causing dental caries: Streptococcus mutans, Streptococcus salivarius,

Streptococcus mitis, and Streptococcus sanguis: an in vitro study. Indian J Dent Res. 2007;18(4):148–51.
75. Nagini S. Neem limonoids as anticancer agents: modulation of cancer hallmarks and oncogenic signaling. Enzyme. 2014;36:131–47.
76. Elmarzugi NA, Elmarzugi NA. A review of chemical constituents and traditional usage of neem plant. Azadirachta Indica. Available from: https://www.academia.edu/35244534/A_Review_of_chemical_constituents_and_traditional_usage_of_Neem_plant_Azadirachta_Indica. [cited 2019 Apr 22].
77. Schumacher M, Cerella C, Reuter S, Dicato M, Diederich M. Anti-inflammatory, pro-apoptotic, and anti-proliferative effects of a methanolic neem (Azadirachta indica) leaf extract are mediated via modulation of the nuclear factor-κB pathway. Genes Nutr. 2011;6(2):149–60.
78. Kim J, Ochoa M-T, Krutzik SR, Takeuchi O, Uematsu S, Legaspi AJ, et al. Activation of toll-like receptor 2 in acne triggers inflammatory cytokine responses. J Immunol. 2002;169(3):1535–41.
79. Chattopadhyay RR, Chattopadhyay RN, Maitra SK. Possible mechanism of antiinflammatory activity of Azadirachta indica leaf extract. Indian J Pharmacol. 1993;25(2):99.
80. Naik MR, Bhattacharya A, Behera R, Agrawal D, Dehury S, Kumar S. Study of anti-inflammatory effect of neem seed oil (*Azadirachta indica*) on infected albino rats, 2014. [Internet]. Available from: http://www.jhrr.org/article.asp?issn=2394-2010;year=2014;volume=1;issue=3;spage=66;epage=69;aulast=Naik. [cited 2019 Apr 22].
81. Bhowmik D, Yadav J, Tripathi KK, Kumar KPS. Herbal remedies of Azadirachta indica and its medicinal application. J Chem Pharm Res. 2010;2(1):62–72.
82. Buhl T, Sulk M, Nowak P, Buddenkotte J, McDonald I, Aubert J, et al. Molecular and morphological characterization of inflammatory infiltrate in rosacea reveals activation of Th1/Th17 pathways. J Invest Dermatol. 2015;135(9):2198–208.
83. Maragathavalli S, Brindha S, Kaviyarasi S, Annadurai B, Gangwar SK. Antimicrobial activity in leaf extract of neem. IJSN. 2012;3:110–3.
84. Nand P, Drabu S, Gupta RK. Insignificant anti-acne activity of Azadirachta indica leaves and bark. J Pharm Negat Results. 2012;3(1):29.
85. Jain A, Basal E. Inhibition of Propionibacterium acnes-induced mediators of inflammation by Indian herbs. Phytomedicine. 2003;10(1):34–8.

86. Pradhan S, Madke B, Kabra P, Singh AL. Anti-inflammatory and immunomodulatory effects of antibiotics and their use in dermatology. Indian J Dermatol. 2016;61(5):469–81.
87. Miglani A, Manchanda RK. Azadirachta indica in treatment of acne vulgaris--an open-label observational study. [Internet]. Available from: http://www.ijrh.org/article.asp?issn=0974-7168;year=2014;volume=8;issue=4;spage=218;epage=223;aulast=Miglani. [cited 2019 Apr 22].
88. Gandhi M, Lal R, Sankaranarayanan A, Banerjee CK, Sharma PL. Acute toxicity study of the oil from Azadirachta indica seed (neem oil). J Ethnopharmacol. 1988;23(1):39–51.
89. PFAF Plant Database. Viburnum opulus-L. [Internet]. Available from: https://pfaf.org/user/Plant.aspx?LatinName=Viburnum+opulus. [cited 2019 Apr 9].
90. Karaçelik AA, Küçük M, İskefiyeli Z, Aydemir S, De Smet S, Miserez B, et al. Antioxidant components of Viburnum opulus L. determined by on-line HPLC-UV-ABTS radical scavenging and LC-UV-ESI-MS methods. Food Chem. 2015;175:106–14.
91. Kraujalytė V, Venskutonis PR, Pukalskas A, Česonienė L, Daubaras R. Antioxidant properties and polyphenolic compositions of fruits from different European cranberrybush (Viburnum opulus L.) genotypes. Food Chem. 2013;141(4):3695–702.
92. Rop O, Reznicek V, Valsikova M, Jurikova T, Mlcek J, Kramarova D. Antioxidant properties of European cranberrybush fruit (Viburnum opulus var. edule). Molecules. 2010;15(6):4467–77.
93. Sagdic O, Aksoy A, Ozkan G. Evaluation of the antibacterial and antioxidant potentials of cranberry (gilaburu, Viburnum opulus L.) fruit extract. Acta Aliment. 2006;35(4):487–92.
94. Nicholson JA, Darby TD, Jarboe CH. Viopudial, a hypotensive and smooth muscle antispasmodic from Viburnum opulus. Proc Soc Exp Biol Med. 1972;140(2):457–61.
95. Singh H, Kaushish Lily M, Dangwal K. Viburnum mullaha D. DON fruit (Indian cranberry): a potential source of polyphenol with rich antioxidant, anti- elastase, anti-collagenase, and anti-tyrosinase activities. Int J Food Prop. 2016;20(8):1729–39.
96. PFAF Plant Database. Urtica dioica-L. [Internet]. Available from: https://pfaf.org/USER/Plant.aspx?LatinName=Urtica+dioica. [cited 2019 Apr 9].
97. Gülçin I, Küfrevioglu OI, Oktay M, Büyükokuroglu ME. Antioxidant, antimicrobial, antiulcer and analgesic activities of nettle (Urtica dioica L.). J Ethnopharmacol. 2004;90(2–3):205–15.

98. Sökeland J. Combined sabal and urtica extract compared with finasteride in men with benign prostatic hyperplasia: analysis of prostate volume and therapeutic outcome. BJU Int. 2000;86(4):439–42.
99. Koch E. Extracts from fruits of saw palmetto (Sabal serrulata) and roots of stinging nettle (Urtica dioica): viable alternatives in the medical treatment of benign prostatic hyperplasia and associated lower urinary tracts symptoms. Planta Med. 2001;67(6):489–500.
100. Randall C, Randall H, Dobbs F, Hutton C, Sanders H. Randomized controlled trial of nettle sting for treatment of base-of-thumb pain. J R Soc Med. 2000;93(6):305–9.
101. Klingelhoefer S, Obertreis B, Quast S, Behnke B. Antirheumatic effect of IDS 23, a stinging nettle leaf extract, on in vitro expression of T helper cytokines. J Rheumatol. 1999;26(12):2517–22.
102. Roschek B, Fink RC, McMichael M, Alberte RS. Nettle extract (Urtica dioica) affects key receptors and enzymes associated with allergic rhinitis. Phytother Res. 2009;23(7):920–6.
103. Bouchentouf S, Said G, Kambouche N, Kress S. Identification of phenolic compounds from nettle as new candidate inhibitors of main enzymes responsible on type-II diabetes. Curr Drug Discov Technol. 2020;17(2):197–202. https://doi.org/10.2174/1570163815666180829094831.

Chapter 5
Introduction to Essential Oils and Essential Oil Processing

Marit K. Kreidel and Mamta Jhaveri

Introduction

Essential oils are hydrophobic, volatile liquids produced through distillation of plant materials to create concentrated plant extracts [1]. Essential oils retain the fragrance and intrinsic properties of the natural plant. All parts of the plant including flowers, leaves, bark, roots, seeds, wood, or peel can be used to make different essential oils, depending on the desired property. Essential oils must be stored in temperate, sealed containers that are not directly exposed to heat or sunlight to avoid evaporation, oxidation, or alterations in chemical properties.

When essential oils are applied to the skin, trans-epidermal absorption and potency are dependent on many factors of the oil, including lipophilicity, polarity, molecule size, molecular weight, and concentration [2]. Since essential oils are lipophilic liquids, they can enter the stratum corneum through intercellular

M. K. Kreidel
Department of Dermatology, Kaiser Permanente, Irvine, CA, USA

M. Jhaveri (✉)
Johns Hopkins Dermatology, Washington, DC, USA
e-mail: mjhaver1@jhmi.edu

R. N. Rupani, P. A. Lio (eds.), *Integrative Dermatology*,
https://doi.org/10.1007/978-3-030-58954-7_5

spaces into the upper dermis [2]. However, high concentrations can lead to damage of keratinocytes, decrease the integrity of the skin barrier, and lead to increased dermal absorption [2]. To optimize epidermal absorption but decrease irritation and minimize side effects, most essential oils are used in the lowest possible concentration and commonly diluted with a carrier oil.

Many of the essential oils are made through extraction processes of steam distillation, solvent extract, or through cold pressure expression of the aromatic plants. The exact method for a desired essential oil can vary, as certain processing methods can be better suited for different plants. Traditional methods of distillation have the potential for degradation via thermal effects or hydrolysis, thereby leading to an interest in different types of extraction [3]. The exact active ingredients of each essential oil will depend on which species of the plant was used, the plant part used, and the distillation process.

- *Steam distillation*: Early writing of steam distillation dates back 5000 years as a way to prepare floral waters [4]. In ancient Greece and Rome, the process entailed exposing glass bottles of flowers to warming from the sun to separate oil form the solid constituents [5]. Below is how steam distillation is most commonly carried out today:
  - Water is heated into a steam and passed through an alembic container.
  - The plant-laden alembic chamber heats and vaporizes.
  - The vapor with the desired essential oil flows out of the chamber and then subsequently condenses into another chamber.
- *Cold expression*: Cold-pressing, also referred to as expression, is specific to citrus essential oils that can include tangerine, lemon, and orange [3]. Initially, this process was completed via sponge pressing and completed via hand without the need for heat [5].
  - Today, a machine known as a sfumatrice, is utilized to squeeze citrus peels at room temperature to release the essential oil [5].
  - The oils are then washed in cold water and isolated via decantation or centrifuging.

- *Hydro-distillation* is essentially solvent distillation with water [3]:
  - Plant materials are immersed in water or other solvent.
  - The mixture is heated until boiling in an alembic chamber.
  - The volatile compounds and water/solvent evaporate at the same pressure.
  - The volatile oil and water/solvent condense and are separated due to differences in density.
  - Vacuum distillation can be utilized to aid in separation of the solvent and essential oil [3].
- *Destructive distillation*: this type of essential oil processing is reserved for wood essential oils [3].
  - The wood's bark and roots undergo destruction from high heat, then distill through tar.
  - Resulting oil is obtained after condensation, decantation, and separation.

With the concern of potential solvent impurities and growing interest in environmentally sound extraction processes, new methods have been developed recently, including CO_2 extraction, turbo distillation, ultrasound-assisted extraction, microwave-assisted extraction, instantaneous controlled pressure drop technology, and other solvent-free methods [3]. It is recommended to use organic oils whenever possible, as pesticide residues can become highly concentrated in the oil.

Essential Oils for Acne

Essential oils are commonly used for acne due to their antimicrobial and anti-inflammatory properties [1]. In the Orchard et al. review of essential oils in dermatologic conditions, 88 of the 98 essential oils reviewed demonstrated potential antimicrobial activity against skin flora [6]. Many of the plant extracts utilized contain intrinsic antibiotic activity against *Cutibacterium acnes* and *Staphylococcus aureus*, two of the main bacteria involved in the pathogenesis of acne [7]. Plant immune systems produce potent defense compounds when exposed to stress: one such compound is resveratrol, which demonstrates in vitro antibacterial activity against *Cutibacterium acnes* [8].

Essential Oils for Rosacea

Topical essential oils are used to improve the skin barrier and redness, decrease trans-epidermal water loss, reduce inflammation, decrease vascular growth factors, and target the demodex mite colonization [9]. One difference from acne vulgaris, however, is that rosacea skin is more easily irritated by topical products, and therefore essential oils must be used with greater caution.

Tea Tree Oil (Melaleuca alternifolia)

Distilled from the leaves and terminal branchlets of the Australian tree *Melaleuca alternifolia*, tea tree oil (TTO) has antiseptic and antimicrobial activity via nonspecific cell membrane damage [10]. Tea tree oil contains at least 100 components, the majority being monoterpenes and sesquiterpenes [11]. Although the International Organization for Standardization (ISO) regulates the concentration range for the 15 major TTO terpenes (ISO 4730:2017), there is still significant variation within this accepted range of these constituents. Terpinen-4-ol constitutes ~30% of TTO found in the United States and is thought to play an important role in the oil's antimicrobial activity [11].

In a study of crowdsourced data from 662 online acne patients, the second most common topical treatment for acne was TTO, behind over-the-counter benzoyl peroxide [12]. Several studies on 5% TTO have noted reductions in acne lesion size and numbers, ranging from 23.7% to 62.1% after products were applied for 4–8 weeks [13]. One study concluded that TTO had antibiotic activity against the biofilms of gram-positive bacteria such as *Staphylococcus aureus*, which was then extrapolated to have activity against the skin biofilms produced by *Cutibacterium acnes* [14]. In another review, the tolerability of TTO was similar to other topical treatments such as benzoyl peroxide and erythromycin [13].

Additionally, TTO has been shown to reduce demodex viability in vitro which can be beneficial in rosacea [15]. However, high concentrations of TTO up to 50–100% were needed to achieve these results, which could lead to localized skin irritation.

Tea tree oil is generally well tolerated, with the most common side effects including irritation, burning, stinging, and pruritus at the site of application. Reports of allergic contact dermatitis to TTO are increasing, with a prevalence up to 3.5% of positive patch test reactions performed [15]. Oxidation of TTO increases its allergic potency, making it important to ensure TTO is fresh and stored properly [15]. Patch testing can be performed to 5% oxidized TTO and is part of the standard North American Contact Dermatitis Panel.

An additional consideration is the development of bacterial resistance to the low concentrations of TTO used in over-the-counter cosmetic products. One study found that both methicillin resistant and sensitive *Staphylococcus aureus* exposed to sublethal concentrations of TTO for 72 hours acquired irreversible stress-hardening, requiring higher concentrations of TTO to reach minimum inhibitory concentrations [16]. Bacterial targets also developed a transient resistance to some commonly used topical antibiotics such as mupirocin [16]. Coagulase-negative staphylococcus did not exhibit stress-hardening but also did exhibit a transient decreased sensitivity to other topical antibiotics [16].

Oregon Grape Root Oil (Mahonia aquifolium or Berberis aquifolium)

Known as *Mahonia aquifolium*, this flower has more potential uses beyond serving as Oregon's state flower. Traditionally, this flower is well-known in Chinese medicine for its compound berberine, found in the roots and bark of the plant [17]. Although not well-studied in the treatment of acne or rosacea, one review noted that berberine and jatorrhizine are the two main active ingredients of *Mahonia aquifolium* and exhibit antimicrobial activity against both *Cutibacterium acnes* and *coagulase-negative staphylococcus* [18]. Berberine has also been shown to suppress lipogenesis in sebaceous glands by 63% in vivo via inhibition of 5-lipocygenase and lipid peroxidation in liposomes [19–21].

Pomegranate Seed Oil (Punica granatum)

Also known as *Punica granatum*, pomegranate seed extract contains four main hydrolysable tannins: punicalagin, punicalin, strictinin A, and granatin B, all of which display activity against *Cutibacterium acnes* [22]. In particular, punicalagin and punicalin have significant antibacterial activities and can also regulate keratinocyte proliferation. Punicalagin, strictinin A, and granatin B also display lipase-inhibitory effects, and specifically granatin B decreases expression of inflammatory markers induced by *Cutibacterium acnes* such as cyclooxygenase-2 and prostaglandin E_2 [22]. Pomegranate polyphenols have also been shown to decrease the expression of interleukin-8 (IL-8) and tumor necrosis factor (TNF)-α production [23].

Rosemary Oil (Rosmarinus officinalis)

Oil extracted from this savory herb has antioxidant, anti-inflammatory, and antimicrobial properties [24, 25]. The main bioactive constituents are rosmarinic acid, carnosol, and carnosic acid. These have been shown to inhibit toll-like receptor-mediated inflammatory responses mediated by lipopolysaccharides [24, 26]. In one study rosemary extract also suppressed the expression of nuclear-factor-kappa-B and proinflammatory cytokines such as IL-8, IL-1β, and TNF-α

from monocytic T1 helper cells when stimulated by *Cutibacterium acnes* [23].

Witch Hazel (Hamamelis virginiana)

This common over-the-counter remedy is extracted from the leaves and bark of *Hamamelis virginiana* and contains the main ingredients of calcium oxalate, gallotannins, safrole, carvacrol, and eugenol [27]. Produced by steam distillation, witch hazel is not technically an essential oil, as it is not volatile at room temperature, but several of its components have essential oil-like properties. Its high tannin content makes it an astringent commonly used for oily skin [28]. Carvacrol has strong antioxidant activity through scavenging reactive oxygen and nitrogen species and is additionally found in oregano oil [29–32]. While not extensively studied to have antimicrobial activity, witch hazel has opportunities as a treatment for cutaneous inflammation [33].

Rose (Rosa damascene)

Extracted from the petals of the damask rose, *Rosa damascene* essential oil extract has exhibited anti-inflammatory, antimicrobial, and antioxidant activity and can also inhibit lipid peroxidation [34]. Studies have shown that *R. damascene* extract has specific antimicrobial activity against *Cutibacterium acnes* and staphylococcus strains, suggesting a need for further research and possible therapeutic benefit of rose essential oil in the treatment of acne and rosacea [35].

Rosehip Oil (Rosa canina)

Rosehip or rosehip seed oil is made from the seeds of *Rosa canina* and is well-known for its antioxidant properties [36]. One of the active ingredients in rosehip oil is α-tocopherol, or vitamin E [37]. In a clinical study, α-tocopherol was tested in conjunction with glycolic acid and found to prevent the formation of atrophic scars in patients with acne vulgaris [38]. A review article on topical vitamins highlighted α-tocopherol's effectiveness against inflammatory dermatoses such as acne [39]. When α-tocopherol was studied in conjunction with benzoyl peroxide, the vitamin had a protective effect against benzoyl peroxide cytotoxicity, suggesting a potential use to help reduce skin irritation [40]. It is important to note, however, that the concentration of α-tocopherol can vary between different rose hip oils based on plants used and extraction methods. In addition, although the rose hip extract anecdotally has antimicrobial activity, this has not been specifically demonstrated against *Cutibacterium acnes* [41]. Although data is limited on the benefit of rosehip oil in acne and rosacea, as a natural source of vitamin E, provitamin A and lipids, it has potential benefit against inflammation and in skin barrier regeneration.

Orange/Citrus Oil

While many types of citrus fruit are available, the most extensively studied citrus essential oils include Korean *Citrus obovoides* and *Citrus natsudaidai*, which reduce *Cutibacterium acnes* induced secretion of interleukin-8 (IL-8) and tumor necrosis factor alpha (TNF-α) [42]. *Citrus medica limonum* (lemon oil) and *Citrus paradisi* (grapefruit) demonstrate antimicrobial activity against *Cutibacterium acnes* specifically [43]. Further investigations into the activity of citrus oils identified limonene and myrcene as common agents in the composition of these fruit essential oils, with particular antimicrobial activity against *Staphylococcus epidermidis* [42–44]. While the bitter orange essential oil *Citrus aurantium* has demonstrated antimicrobial activity in in vitro studies, it is not well studied in clinical studies [6].

Citrus essential oils can be phototoxic and increase photosensitivity, especially at higher concentrations [45]. Therefore, it is often recommended to use these at night and wash them off in the morning.

Korean Fir (Abies koreana)

This lesser known essential oil has been found to have excellent anti-inflammatory and antibacterial activities against cutaneous microbes. One study identified the major components of *Korean fir* essential oil as bornyl acetate (30%) and limonene (19%) [46]. *Abies koreana* showed excellent antibacterial activities against drug-susceptible and resistant *Cutibacterium acnes* and *Staphylococcus epidermidis* [47]. This reduction in bacterial load reduced the secretion of lipopolysaccharide-induced secretion of tumor necrosis factor-alpha (TNF-alpha), interleukin-1beta (IL-1β), interleukin-6 (IL-6), nitrous oxide (NO), and prostaglandin-E2 (PGE-2) [46].

Frankincense Oil (Boswellia carterii)

Frankincense (*boswellia*) belongs to the family Burseraceae and is steam distilled from the gum/resin of the Somalia/Yemen plant. It is also known as "olibanum," but the word frankincense is derived from the French word for "real incense." It has been used in religious ceremonies for hundreds of years. In ancient times, it was valued more than gold, due to its healing and anointing powers [48]. The composition is mostly monoterpenes followed by sesquiterpenes and monoterpenols. In a 2007 study, *Boswellia* extract was shown to be effective against *Cutibacterium acnes*, *Clostridium perfringens*, and *Porphyromonas gingivalis* at low concentrations [49, 50]. In a follow-up study, *Boswellia* extract was also shown to have antimicrobial activity against *Malassezia* species, *Candida*, and *Trichophyton* [51].

Chamomile (Anthemis aciphylla discoidea)

Chamomile has long been used to treat skin inflammation, and it has been noted to have the same anti-inflammatory effect as hydrocortisone 0.25–1% [52]. Most of the literature for chamomile in skin disease centers around eczema, but it is a great option to soothe the redness in acne and rosacea. Creams or ointments should contain 20 g of the essential oil for every 100 g of vehicle or carrier oil. Chamomile baths or compresses are a popular option: 6 g of dried chamomile powdered flower heads are diluted into 150 g of water. A washcloth can be soaked and then applied to affected skin for 1 hour twice a day [52].

Patients who are allergic to the Compositae family (chrysanthemum, aster, daisy, sunflower, dandelion, *Echinacea*) should not use chamomile due to the high risk of allergic contact dermatitis.

Clary Sage (Salvia sclarea)

Clary sage belongs to the family *Lamiaceae* and is steam distilled from the flowering plant. It has long been used as an eye wash and to treat skin infections. It is known to calm and soothe the skin and reduce inflammation [48].

In a study conducted at an academic medical center, 61 patients with resistant staphylococcal wounds underwent bacterial culture and susceptibility testing to clary sage extract. Of these 61 patients, there were 11 different MRSA strains and 16 different MSSA strains; all of them were resistant to penicillin. The clary sage oil showed antimicrobial activity against all of these strains with MIC between 3.75 and 7.00 μL/mL [53]. Clary sage has more than 56 constituents, and those in the highest concentration are linalyl acetate and linalool. The constituents that were present in significant concentrations with the lowest MIC were a-pinene, b-pinene, and sabinene [53]. Owing to this antibacterial and anti-inflammatory property of clary sage, it has been incorporated into commercially available skincare products.

Patients who are allergic to the linalool should not use clary sage given the high risk of allergic contact dermatitis, although cases of contact dermatitis to clary sage have yet to be reported.

Lavender Oil (Lavandula angustifolia and latifolia)

Lavender also belongs to the *Lamiaceae* family, and the essential oil is produced by steam distillation of the flowering tops. The major constituents are linalyl butyrate and linalool. Lavender essential oil can be used for both acne and rosacea due to its antimicrobial, antioxidant, and stress reduction properties. There are a few reports of its antimicrobial activity against gram-positive bacteria such as *Staphylococcus aureus* [50]. A study also found that topical application of lavender oil accelerated wound healing by promoting collagen synthesis and upregulation of tumor growth factor-β [54].

Application or inhalation of lavender oil induces relaxation and reduces stress [47]. Stress can precipitate flares in both acne and rosacea, and, therefore, it is believed that application of lavender oil to pulse points or soles of the feet can indirectly improve acne and rosacea flares [47].

Lavender oil and linalool can cause an allergic contact dermatitis in sensitized patients. Given the diversity of lavender constituents, it is difficult to consistently perform patch testing to confirm reactivity to lavender oil [55].

Ylang-Ylang Oil (Cananga odorata)

Ylang-ylang oil is produced by steam distillation from the fragrant flower of the tree. Although there are many active ingredients in ylang-ylang oil, the main chemical components are linalool and two sesquiterpenes, germacrene, and caryophyllene [56]. Ylang-ylang essential oil was shown to have antimicrobial activity against *Staphylococcus aureus* and *Cutibacterium acnes* and also able to disrupt their biofilm [56]. It also exhibited anti-inflammatory and antioxidant properties, including strong inhibition of lipoxygenase [56]. Ylang-ylang oil can cause contact dermatitis and should be avoided in patients allergic to linalool or other sesquiterpenes.

Juniper Berry Oil (Juniperus communis)

Juniper berry oil is produced by steam distillation of the berries of the juniper evergreen tree. The major component of juniper oil is α-pinene. Juniper berry oil has been found to have strong antioxidant and antimicrobial activity against methicillin-resistant and methicillin-sensitive *Staphylococcus aureus* [57].

Clove Basil (Ocimum gratissimum)

Ocimum gratissimum oil produced from the leaves of the plant has been studied in the treatment of acne. The major active component is eugenol, which can be an antimicrobial agent due to membrane disruption [58]. When *Ocimum gratissimum* oil was formulated in a cetomacrogol blend base, it was more effective than 10% benzoyl peroxide lotion in treating acne lesions [59]. When combined with aloe vera gel, the basil essential oil was more effective than topical 1% clindamycin [60]. Another study investigating Thai basil oils *O. basilicum* and *O. sanctum* demonstrated potential for acne treatment due to the antimicrobial activity against *Cutibacterium acnes* [61].

Topical Application of Essential Oils

While some essential oils can be applied directly to the skin, most should be diluted with a carrier oil to decrease skin irritation or allergic reaction. Carrier oils are fixed oils, meaning they are not volatile at room temperature. When added to an essential oil, they help allow the essential oil to penetrate the surface of skin. While the carrier oils are comprised of various fatty acids and triglycerides, the fatty acid linoleic acid helps maintain the water permeability barrier of the skin [62]. Carrier oils with a higher linoleic acid to oleic acid ratio had improved repair potential, whereas oils with higher concentrations of oleic acid could be irritating and harmful to the skin-barrier function [63]. In assessment of specific oils, cold-pressing was the preferred method of extracting the oil, with decreased byproducts [63]. The most popular carrier oils are olive (*Olea europaea*), jojoba (*Simmondsia chinensis*), coconut (*Coco nucifera*), sesame seed (*Sesamum indicum*), grape seed (*Vitis vinifera*), sweet almond (*Amygdalus dulcis*), and sunflower seed (*Helianthus annuus*) oil.

To mix an essential oil with a carrier oil, it is recommended to use a glass bottle, preferably dark or amber colored. It is important to store the oils at a cool temperature and away from direct light. One to three drops of these essential oils can be mixed with a carrier oil to help make washes, serums, and spot treatment for acne and rosacea. If the oil is applied directly to the skin, it is recommended to use a clean cotton ball with one to three drops of the oil spread evenly over the acne affected area.

Carrier Oil: Olive Oil (Olea europaea)

One of the most well-known oils, particularly for dietary consumption as well as topical application, olive oil consists mostly of oleic acid with decent amounts of linoleic acid and palmitic acid [64]. The majority of the studies of olive oil are in regard to dietary consumption, and the high concentration of oleic acid may enable greater depth of skin barrier penetration but could lead to skin irritation and inflammation.

Carrier Oil: Jojoba Oil (Simmondsia chinensis)

Obtained from drought-resistant plants, this carrier oil has wax esters and is commonly used in commercial moisturizers and sunscreens, as well as to enhance the absorption of topical drugs [65]. In a study investigating its potential therapeutic actions with tazarotene, jojoba oil helped reduce inflammation and irritation [66]. While the study investigated its use for psoriasis, given that tazarotene has acne applications, jojoba oil could be utilized as a soothing adjuvant therapy when combined with a traditional acne treatment regimen.

Carrier Oil: Coconut Oil (Cocos nucifera)

While known for its moisturizing properties, this carrier oil has also been studied for its anti-inflammatory potential against UVB-induced inflammation as well as increased collagen and hyaluronan synthase-3 expression [67]. In a study examining coconut oil on delicate neonatal skin, topically applied coconut oil had no adverse effects, particularly in preterm infants [68]. The potential therapies of coconut oil center around its high composition of polyphenols and fatty acids [67]. In addition, monolaurin, which is one of the major fatty acid components of coconut oil and is derived from lauric acid, has antibacterial activity against *Cutibacterium acnes*, *Staphylococcus aureus*, and *Staphylococcus epidermidis* [69].

Carrier Oil: Sesame Seed Oil (Sesamum indicum)

The active components of sesame oil are sesamin, sesamolin, and sesaminol, which exhibit antioxidant activity [70]. In animal studies, sesame oil showed potential promise for antioxidant activity via inhibiting the production of xanthine oxidase and nitric oxide [71]. An additional study investigating the effects of topical sesame oil showed potential protective effects against ultraviolet radiation, but further evidence-based studies are needed to determine the efficacy of sesame oil as a treatment option [72].

Carrier Oil: Grape Seed/Grape Vine (Vitis vinifera)

Known scientifically as *Vitis vinifera*, this Mediterranean plant extract has growth inhibitory activity. One study also noted that grape-seed oil may partially eradicate a mature *Cutibacterium acnes* biofilm [73, 74]. The inhibitory activity by grape-seed extract can be attributed to horizontal inter-kingdom of the opportunistic pathogen *Cutibacterium acnes* with the grape-seed crop [75].

Carrier Oil: Sweet Almond Oil (Amygdalus amygdalae)

This popular nut also has potential to moisturize skin and potentially prevent DNA structural damage caused by UV radiation [76]. With regard to acne and rosacea, its benefit is primarily in the category of a carrier oil.

Carrier Oil: Sunflower Seed Oil (Helianthus annuus)

Due to this oil's high ratio of linoleic acid to oleic acid, sunflower seed oil enhances the skin barrier and has been shown to preserve stratum corneum integrity, as well as improve skin hydration without inducing erythema [77]. The active properties of linoleic acid are attributed to activation of the peroxisome proliferator-activated receptor-alpha (PPAR-α), which then enhances lipid synthesis through keratinocyte proliferation [77]. Additional studies have examined sunflower seed oil on neonatal skin, but these few studies have limited long-term implications and significant evidence-based support.

With all variations of names and spellings, too often the specific essential oils can be lost in translation. Presented here are essential oils and their common names, as well as characteristics of each oil (Table 5.1).

TABLE 5.1 Summary of commonly used topical essential oils and their active properties

Common name	Botanical name	Active compound	Properties
Tea tree oil	*Melaleuca alternifolia*	Terpenes	Antimicrobial via nonspecific cell membrane damage
Oregon grape root oil	*Mahonia aquifolium or Berberis aquifolium*	Berberine and Jatorrhizine	Antimicrobial, decreased lipogenesis
Pomegranate seed oil	*Punica granatum*	Punicalagin, punicalin, strinin A, granatin	Antimicrobial, UV protective, regulates keratinocyte proliferation and inhibits lipase activity
Rosemary oil	*Rosmarinus officinalis*	Rosmarinic acid, carnosol, carnosic acid	Antimicrobial, anti-inflammatory
Witch hazel	*Hamamelis virginiana*	Calcium oxalate, gallotannins, safrole, carvacrol, eugenol	Astringent
Rose	*Rosa damascene*	Very varied dependent on the species	Antimicrobial, anti-inflammatory, anti-oxidant
Rosehip oil	*Rosa canina*	alpha-tocopherol, provitamin A	Anti-inflammatory, antioxidant
Orange/citrus oil	*Citrus obovoides and natsudaidai*	Limonene, myrcene	Anti-inflammatory, antioxidant

TABLE 5.1 (continued)

Common name	Botanical name	Active compound	Properties
Korean fir	*Abies koreana*	Bornyl acetate, limonene	Antimicrobial
Frankincense oil	*Boswellia carterii*	Terpenes, monoterpenols	Antimicrobial
Chamomile	*Anthemis aciphylla discoidea*	–	Anti-inflammatory, soothing
Clary Sage	*Salvia sclarea*	Linalyl acetate, linalool	Antimicrobial, anti-inflammatory
Lavender	*Lavandula angustifolia and latifolia*	Linalool, linalyl-butyrate	Antimicrobial, anti-stress
Ylang-ylang oil	*Cananga odorata*	Linalool, germacrene, caryophyllene	Antimicrobial, anti-inflammatory
Juniper berry oil	*Juniperus communis*	α-Pinene	Antimicrobial
Clove basil oil	*Ocimum gratissimum*	Eugenol and myrcene	Antimicrobial via cell membrane disruption

Conclusion

As the range of topical therapies for the treatment of acne and rosacea continues to broaden, essential oils such as tea tree oil can serve as promising treatment options. This chapter has summarized the evidence behind commonly used essential oils and their carrier oils to guide decisions for providers and patients with acne and rosacea. Primarily for their antimicrobial, anti-inflammatory and antioxidative potential, essential oils are gaining popularity, but further double-blinded trials regarding effective use are required.

References

1. Winkelman WJ. Aromatherapy, botanicals, and essential oils in acne. Clin Dermatol. 2018;36(3):299–305.
2. Herman A, Herman AP. Essential oils and their constituents as skin penetration enhancer for transdermal drug delivery: a review. J Pharm Pharmacol. 2015;7(4):473–85.
3. Li Y, Fabiano-Tixier A-S, Chemat F. Essential oils: from conventional to green extraction. In: Essential oils as reagents in green chemistry. Cham: Springer; 2014. p. 9–20.
4. Schnaubelt K. Biology of essential oils. San Rafael: Terra Linda Scent and Image; 2002.
5. Guenther E. The essential oils. New York: D. Van Nostrand Company, Inc.; 1948.
6. Orchard A, van Vuuren S. Commercial essential oils as potential antimicrobials to treat skin diseases. Evid Based Complement Alternat Med. 2017;2017:4517971.
7. Olutunmbi Y, Paley K, English JC 3rd. Adolescent female acne: etiology and management. J Pediatr Adolesc Gynecol. 2008;21(4):171–6.
8. Taylor EJ, Yu Y, Champer J, Kim J. Resveratrol demonstrates antimicrobial effects against propionibacterium acnes in vitro. Dermatol Ther. 2014;4(2):249–57.
9. Fisk WA, Lev-Tov HA, Sivamani RK. Botanical and phytochemical therapy of acne: a systematic review. Phytother Res. 2014;28(8):1137–52.
10. Carson CF, Mee BJ, Riley TV. Mechanism of action of Melaleuca alternifolia (tea tree) oil on Staphylococcus aureus determined by time-kill, lysis, leakage, and salt tolerance assays and electron microscopy. Antimicrob Agents Chemother. 2002;46(6):1914–20.
11. Sharifi-Rad J, Salehi B, Varoni EM, Sharopov F, Yousaf Z, Ayatollahi SA, et al. Plants of the Melaleuca genus as antimicrobial agents: from farm to pharmacy. Phytother Res. 2017;31(10):1475–94.

12. Armstrong AW, Cheeney S, Wu J, Harskamp CT, Schupp CW. Harnessing the power of crowds: crowdsourcing as a novel research method for evaluation of acne treatments. Am J Clin Dermatol. 2012;13(6):405–16.
13. Hammer KA. Treatment of acne with tea tree oil (melaleuca) products: a review of efficacy, tolerability and potential modes of action. Int J Antimicrob Agents. 2015;45(2):106–10.
14. Brady A, Loughlin R, Gilpin D, Kearney P, Tunney M. In vitro activity of tea-tree oil against clinical skin isolates of meticillin-resistant and -sensitive Staphylococcus aureus and coagulase-negative staphylococci growing planktonically and as biofilms. J Med Microbiol. 2006;55(Pt 10):1375–80.
15. de Groot AC, Schmidt E. Tea tree oil: contact allergy and chemical composition. Contact Dermatitis. 2016;75(3):129–43.
16. McMahon M, Tunney M, Moore J, Blair I, Gilpin D, McDowell D. Changes in antibiotic susceptibility in staphylococci habituated to sub-lethal concentrations of tea tree oil (Melaleuca alternifolia). Lett Appl Microbiol. 2008;47(4):263–8.
17. He JM, Mu Q. The medicinal uses of the genus Mahonia in traditional Chinese medicine: an ethnopharmacological, phytochemical and pharmacological review. J Ethnopharmacol. 2015;175:668–83.
18. Slobodnikova L, Kost'alova D, Labudova D, Kotulova D, Kettmann V. Antimicrobial activity of Mahonia aquifolium crude extract and its major isolated alkaloids. Phytother Res. 2004;18(8):674–6.
19. Gulliver WP, Donsky HJ. A report on three recent clinical trials using Mahonia aquifolium 10% topical cream and a review of the worldwide clinical experience with Mahonia aquifolium for the treatment of plaque psoriasis. Am J Ther. 2005;12(5):398–406.
20. Muller K, Ziereis K. The antipsoriatic Mahonia aquifolium and its active constituents; I. Pro- and antioxidant properties and inhibition of 5-lipoxygenase. Planta Med. 1994;60(5):421–4.
21. Misik V, Bezakova L, Malekova L, Kostalova D. Lipoxygenase inhibition and antioxidant properties of protoberberine and aporphine alkaloids isolated from Mahonia aquifolium. Planta Med. 1995;61(4):372–3.
22. Lee CJ, Chen LG, Liang WL, Wang CC. Multiple activities of Punica granatum linne against acne vulgaris. Int J Mol Sci. 2017;18(1):141.
23. Tsai TH, Chuang LT, Lien TJ, Liing YR, Chen WY, Tsai PJ. Rosmarinus officinalis extract suppresses Propionibacterium

acnes-induced inflammatory responses. J Med Food. 2013;16(4):324–33.
24. Peng CH, Su JD, Chyau CC, Sung TY, Ho SS, Peng CC, et al. Supercritical fluid extracts of rosemary leaves exhibit potent anti-inflammation and anti-tumor effects. Biosci Biotechnol Biochem. 2007;71(9):2223–32.
25. Baumann LS. Less-known botanical cosmeceuticals. Dermatol Ther. 2007;20(5):330–42.
26. Cheung S, Tai J. Anti-proliferative and antioxidant properties of rosemary Rosmarinus officinalis. Oncol Rep. 2007;17(6):1525–31.
27. Council of Europe. Natural sources of flavourings. Report No 3, 2008. Available from: https://book.coe.int/en/health-protection-of-the-consumer/4006-natural-sources-of-flavourings-report-no-3.html.
28. Chularojanamontri L, Tuchinda P, Kulthanan K, Pongparit K. Moisturizers for acne: what are their constituents? J Clin Aesthet Dermatol. 2014;7(5):36–44.
29. Sheibani V, Afarinesh M, Hajializadeh Z, Abbasnejad M, Haghpanah T, Arabnezhad R, et al. Evaluation of Origanum vulgare L. ssp. viridis leaves extract effect on discrimination learning and ltp induction in the ca1 region of the rat hippocampus. Iran J Basic Med Sci. 2011;14(2):177–84.
30. Yang R, Shetty K. Stimulation of Rosmarinic acid in shoot cultures of oregano (Origanum vulgare) clonal line in response to proline, proline analogue, and proline precursors. J Agric Food Chem. 1998;46(7):2888–93.
31. Lambert RJ, Skandamis PN, Coote PJ, Nychas GJ. A study of the minimum inhibitory concentration and mode of action of oregano essential oil, thymol and carvacrol. J Appl Microbiol. 2001;91(3):453–62.
32. Coccimiglio J, Alipour M, Jiang ZH, Gottardo C, Suntres Z. Antioxidant, antibacterial, and cytotoxic activities of the ethanolic Origanum vulgare extract and its major constituents. Oxidative Med Cell Longev. 2016;2016:1404505.
33. Colantonio S, Rivers JK. Botanicals with dermatologic properties derived from first nations healing: part 2-plants and algae. J Cutan Med Surg. 2017;21(4):299–307.
34. Shahriari S, Yasa N, Mohammadirad A, Khorasani R, Abdollahi M. In vivo antioxidant potentials of Rosa damascene petal extract from Guilan, Iran, comparable to alpha-tocopherol. Int J Pharmacol. 2007;3(2):187–90.

35. Hajhashemi V, Ghannadi A, Hajiloo M. Analgesic and anti-inflammatory effects of Rosa damascena hydroalcoholic extract and its essential oil in animal models. Iran J Pharm Res. 2010;9(2):163–8.
36. Jimenez S, Gascon S, Luquin A, Laguna M, Ancin-Azpilicueta C, Rodriguez-Yoldi MJ. Rosa canina extracts have antiproliferative and antioxidant effects on Caco-2 human colon cancer. PLoS One. 2016;11(7):e0159136.
37. Andersson SC, Olsson ME, Gustavsson KE, Johansson E, Rumpunen K. Tocopherols in rose hips (Rosa spp.) during ripening. J Sci Food Agric. 2012;92(10):2116–21.
38. Kurokawa I, Oiso N, Kawada A. Adjuvant alternative treatment with chemical peeling and subsequent iontophoresis for postinflammatory hyperpigmentation, erosion with inflamed red papules and non-inflamed atrophic scars in acne vulgaris. J Dermatol. 2017;44(4):401–5.
39. Burgess C. Topical vitamins. J Drugs Dermatol. 2008;7(7 Suppl):s2–6.
40. Bellei E, Rota C, Bergamini S, Manfredini P, Albertazzi A, Tomasi A, et al. Effect of alpha-tocopherol and N-acetylcysteine on benzoyl peroxide toxicity in human keratinocytes. J Biochem Mol Toxicol. 2004;18(2):107–14.
41. Marmol I, Sanchez-de-Diego C, Jimenez-Moreno N, Ancin-Azpilicueta C, Rodriguez-Yoldi MJ. Therapeutic applications of rose hips from different rosa species. Int J Mol Sci. 2017;18(6):1137.
42. Kim SS, Baik JS, Oh TH, Yoon WJ, Lee NH, Hyun CG. Biological activities of Korean citrus obovoides and citrus natsudaidai essential oils against acne-inducing bacteria. Biosci Biotechnol Biochem. 2008;72(10):2507–13.
43. Zu Y, Yu H, Liang L, Fu Y, Efferth T, Liu X, et al. Activities of ten essential oils towards Propionibacterium acnes and PC-3, A-549 and MCF-7 cancer cells. Molecules. 2010;15(5):3200–10.
44. Baik JS, Kim SS, Lee JA, Oh TH, Kim JY, Lee NH, et al. Chemical composition and biological activities of essential oils extracted from Korean endemic citrus species. J Microbiol Biotechnol. 2008;18(1):74–9.
45. Naganuma M, Hirose S, Nakayama Y, Nakajima K, Someya T. A study of the phototoxicity of lemon oil. Arch Dermatol Res. 1985;278(1):31–6.
46. Yoon WJ, Kim SS, Oh TH, Lee NH, Hyun CG. Abies koreana essential oil inhibits drug-resistant skin pathogen growth

and LPS-induced inflammatory effects of murine macrophage. Lipids. 2009;44(5):471–6.
47. Sayorwan W, Siripornpanich V, Piriyapunyaporn T, Hongratanaworakit T, Kotchabhakdi N, Ruangrungsi N. The effects of lavender oil inhalation on emotional states, autonomic nervous system, and brain electrical activity. J Med Assoc Thail. 2012;95(4):598–606.
48. Essential Science Publishing. Essential oils desk reference. Orem: Essential Science Publishing; 2014.
49. Weckesser S, Engel K, Simon-Haarhaus B, Wittmer A, Pelz K, Schempp C. Screening of plant extracts for antimicrobial activity against bacteria and yeasts with dermatological relevance. Phytomedicine. 2007;14(7–8):508–16.
50. Man A, Santacroce L, Jacob R, Mare A, Man L. Antimicrobial activity of six essential oils against a group of human pathogens: a comparative study. Pathogens. 2019;8(1):15.
51. Sadhasivam S, Palanivel S, Ghosh S. Synergistic antimicrobial activity of Boswellia serrata Roxb. ex Colebr.(Burseraceae) essential oil with various azoles against pathogens associated with skin, scalp and nail infections. Lett Appl Microbiol. 2016;63(6):495–501.
52. Charousaei F, Dabirian A, Mojab F. Using chamomile solution or a 1% topical hydrocortisone ointment in the management of peristomal skin lesions in colostomy patients: results of a controlled clinical study. Ostomy Wound Manage. 2011;57(5):28.
53. Sienkiewicz M, Głowacka A, Poznańska-Kurowska K, Kaszuba A, Urbaniak A, Kowalczyk E. The effect of clary sage oil on staphylococci responsible for wound infections. Postepy Dermatol Alergol. 2015;32(1):21–6.
54. Mori H-M, Kawanami H, Kawahata H, Aoki M. Wound healing potential of lavender oil by acceleration of granulation and wound contraction through induction of TGF-β in a rat model. BMC Complement Altern Med. 2016;16(1):144.
55. Bingham LJ, Tam MM, Palmer AM, Cahill JL, Nixon RL. Contact allergy and allergic contact dermatitis to lavender: a retrospective study from an Australian clinic. Contact Dermatitis. 2019;81(1):37–42.
56. Tan LTH, Lee LH, Yin WF, Chan CK, Abdul Kadir H, Chan KG, et al. Traditional uses, phytochemistry, and bioactivities of Cananga odorata (Ylang-Ylang). Evid Based Complement Alternat Med. 2015;2015:896314.

57. Filipowicz N, Kamiński M, Kurlenda J, Asztemborska M, Ochocka JR. Antibacterial and antifungal activity of juniper berry oil and its selected components. Phytother Res. 2003;17(3):227–31.
58. Chimnoi N, Reuk-ngam N, Chuysinuan P, Khlaychan P, Khunnawutmanotham N, Chokchaichamnankit D, et al. Characterization of essential oil from Ocimum gratissimum leaves: antibacterial and mode of action against selected gastroenteritis pathogens. Microb Pathog. 2018;118:290–300.
59. Orafidiya L, Agbani E, Oyedele A, Babalola O, Onayemi O. Preliminary clinical tests on topical preparations of Ocimum gratissimum Linn leaf essential oil for the treatment of acne vulgaris. Clin Drug Investig. 2002;22(5):313–9.
60. Orafidiya L, Agbani E, Oyedele A, Babalola O, Onayemi O, Aiyedun F. The effect of aloe vera gel on the anti-acne properties of the essential oil of Ocimum gratissimum Linn leaf–a preliminary clinical investigation. Int J Aromather. 2004;14(1):15–21.
61. Viyoch J, Pisutthanan N, Faikreua A, Nupangta K, Wangtorpol K, Ngokkuen J. Evaluation of in vitro antimicrobial activity of Thai basil oils and their micro-emulsion formulas against Propionibacterium acnes. Int J Cosmet Sci. 2006;28(2):125–33.
62. Elias PM, Brown BE, Ziboh VA. The permeability barrier in essential fatty acid deficiency: evidence for a direct role for linoleic acid in barrier function. J Invest Dermatol. 1980;74(4):230–3.
63. Vaughn AR, Clark AK, Sivamani RK, Shi VY. Natural oils for skin-barrier repair: ancient compounds now backed by modern science. Am J Clin Dermatol. 2018;19(1):103–17.
64. Lin TK, Zhong L, Santiago JL. Anti-inflammatory and skin barrier repair effects of topical application of some plant oils. Int J Mol Sci. 2017;19(1):70.
65. Pazyar N, Yaghoobi R, Ghassemi MR, Kazerouni A, Rafeie E, Jamshydian N. Jojoba in dermatology: a succinct review. G Ital Dermatol Venereol. 2013;148(6):687–91.
66. Nasr M, Abdel-Hamid S, Moftah NH, Fadel M, Alyoussef AA. Jojoba oil soft colloidal nanocarrier of a synthetic retinoid: preparation, characterization and clinical efficacy in psoriatic patients. Curr Drug Deliv. 2017;14(3):426–32.
67. Kim S, Jang JE, Kim J, Lee YI, Lee DW, Song SY, et al. Enhanced barrier functions and anti-inflammatory effect of cultured coconut extract on human skin. Food Chem Toxicol. 2017;106(Pt A):367–75.
68. Strunk T, Pupala S, Hibbert J, Doherty D, Patole S. Topical coconut oil in very preterm infants: an open-label randomised controlled trial. Neonatology. 2018;113(2):146–51.

69. Preuss HG, Echard B, Enig M, Brook I, Elliott TB. Minimum inhibitory concentrations of herbal essential oils and monolaurin for gram-positive and gram-negative bacteria. Mol Cell Biochem. 2005;272(1–2):29–34.
70. Dar AA, Arumugam N. Lignans of sesame: purification methods, biological activities and biosynthesis – a review. Bioorg Chem. 2013;50:1–10.
71. Chiang JP, Hsu DZ, Tsai JC, Sheu HM, Liu MY. Effects of topical sesame oil on oxidative stress in rats. Altern Ther Health Med. 2005;11(6):40–5.
72. Korac RR, Khambholja KM. Potential of herbs in skin protection from ultraviolet radiation. Pharmacogn Rev. 2011;5(10):164–73.
73. Nelson K, Lyles JT, Li T, Saitta A, Addie-Noye E, Tyler P, et al. Anti-acne activity of Italian medicinal plants used for skin infection. Front Pharmacol. 2016;7:425.
74. Coenye T, Brackman G, Rigole P, De Witte E, Honraet K, Rossel B, et al. Eradication of Propionibacterium acnes biofilms by plant extracts and putative identification of icariin, resveratrol and salidroside as active compounds. Phytomedicine. 2012;19(5):409–12.
75. Campisano A, Ometto L, Compant S, Pancher M, Antonielli L, Yousaf S, et al. Interkingdom transfer of the acne-causing agent, Propionibacterium acnes, from human to grapevine. Mol Biol Evol. 2014;31(5):1059–65.
76. Sultana Y, Kohli K, Athar M, Khar RK, Aqil M. Effect of pre-treatment of almond oil on ultraviolet B-induced cutaneous photoaging in mice. J Cosmet Dermatol. 2007;6(1):14–9.
77. Danby SG, AlEnezi T, Sultan A, Lavender T, Chittock J, Brown K, et al. Effect of olive and sunflower seed oil on the adult skin barrier: implications for neonatal skin care. Pediatr Dermatol. 2013;30(1):42–50.

Chapter 6
Bee Products

Neha Chandan and Sara Dill

Introduction

Apitherapy is a branch of complementary and alternative medicine that uses naturally derived bee products, including those of honey, propolis, and bee venom, for their potential health benefits. Given their increasing popularity in skin care, clinical studies have been and are being performed to investigate the use of bee products in common skin conditions, including acne and rosacea. In this chapter, we will provide a review of the current literature focusing on the potential efficacy of honey, propolis, and bee venom in the treatment of acne and rosacea, discuss how they compare to today's standard medical therapeutic options, as well as discuss potential side effects, risks, and harms that one ought to be aware of when using or recommending these agents.

N. Chandan (✉)
Department of Dermatology, University of Illinois Hospital & Health Sciences System, Chicago, IL, USA

S. Dill
Luminous Dermatology, Santa Barbara, CA, USA

R. N. Rupani, P. A. Lio (eds.), *Integrative Dermatology*,
https://doi.org/10.1007/978-3-030-58954-7_6

Honey

Honey is a supersaturated sugary solution derived from the nectar of flowering plants and processed by bees to be broken down into simple sugars, which are then stored in a wax-like structure called honeycomb [1]. A natural antibiotic and anti-inflammatory agent, honey contains many antioxidants, vitamins—including B2, B3, and B5—and minerals [2, 3]. Popularly known to soothe sore throats, honey is paving a path for dermatological uses as well, with current applications including dressing for wounds and burns; treatment against psoriasis, tinea, seborrhea, pityriasis, and diaper dermatitis; and prevention of pathogen infections in the skin [2, 3]. This product is extensively used in cosmetics as well, by exerting soothing, brightening, renewing, and antiaging effects [2]. In fact, of all the bee products used in skin care, honey is perhaps the most popular, affordable, and well-studied, with honey-based products lining the shelves of drug stores and high-end beauty stores alike, in products ranging from lip ointments and hydrating creams to cleansing creams, shampoos, and conditioners [2] (Fig. 6.1).

Many speculations have been made about how exactly honey helps acne, with the current findings summarized in Table 6.1. Treatment modalities include spot treatments,

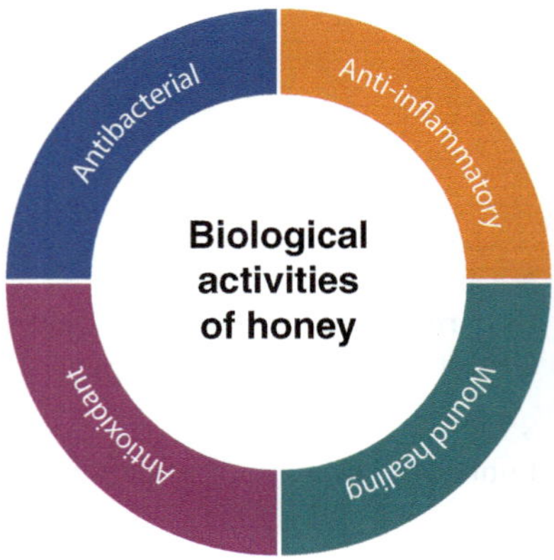

FIGURE 6.1 Biological activities of honey

TABLE 6.1 Topical use of honey in *Acne vulgaris*

Property of honey	Mechanism of effect on acne
Antimicrobial	Fights off bacteria in the skin
Anti-inflammatory	Reduces redness, swelling, and pain associated with acne
Antioxidant	Prevents damage to the skin caused by free radicals in the environment; especially important as acne lesions open and leave the skin exposed and unprotected
Immunostimulatory	Promotes release of tumor necrosis factor-alpha from the immune system to promote the body for fighting and healing
Antiseptic, moisturizing	Facilitates healing of wounds and fades scars created by acne
Low pH (3.4–5.5)	Disrupts optimal, neutral pH of bacteria; creates unfavorable environment for bacterial enzymatic function
High osmolarity due to sugar content	Draws water out of wound and keeps wound surfaces moist for better healing

masks, and cleansers. Apart from topical uses, it has also been hypothesized that consumption of honey can "clean blood" and "boost metabolism," facilitating proper blood circulation to aid in the removal of toxins that can otherwise build up and affect overall skin appearance [4]. Different types of honey seem to have different therapeutic modalities. Herein we will focus on kanuka and manuka honey, two popular honeys derived from New Zealand and used extensively for the treatment of acne and rosacea.

Kanuka Honey

Kanuka honey is honey that bees have produced using the flowers of the kanuka tree (*Kunzea ericoides*), a tree found only in New Zealand [5]. It has been hypothesized that kanuka honey has both more powerful anti-inflammatory and immunostimulatory properties than manuka honey [6–8]. However, its use in acne is still controversial. A 2016 study found that when a topical formulation of 90% medical-grade kanuka honey and 10% glycerine was used in combination with a triclocarban-based antibacterial soap twice daily for 12 weeks, 7.6% of participants had a significant improvement in Investigator Global Assessment (IGA) for acne score (defined as greater than or equal to two grades of improvement), as compared to 1.9% of participants using the antibacterial soap alone [9]. These results demonstrate nearly four times the number of patients showing improvement with the honey combination versus the soap alone, suggesting that there does appear to be an effect beyond the control group (which was in fact not a placebo but an antibacterial soap), although the effect seems to be modest at best. Notably, the trial reports possible concerns regarding treatment adherence amongst the participants. Nonetheless, honey products may still be an option for long-term acne sufferers, as there was moderate evidence for reduction of acne severity and fewer acne lesions [9]. Additionally, there was no difference in adverse events reported between the honey compound users and antibacterial soap-only users, suggesting that honey is relatively safe for the skin, with only mildly irritant effects such as stinging of skin when applied to acne lesions [9].

More promising results have been found for kanuka honey's use in rosacea. A 2015 study brought to light the efficacy of this product, with 34.4% of participants who used the same honey compound for 8 weeks having significant improvement in the severity score of their rosacea (≥2 points on the Investigator Global Assessment of Rosacea Severity Score [IGA-RSS]) [10]. Additionally, the overall relative risk (RR) of improvement was found to be 2.03, with clinical efficacy observed in just 2 weeks of treatment [10]. Similar studies evaluating the efficacy of topical metronidazole in rosacea found an RR of improvement of 1.95, leading some to hypothesize that this honey compound may be more effective than topical metronidazole [11, 12]. However, studies directly comparing kanuka honey to conventional treatments of rosacea, including topical metronidazole and azelaic acid, have not yet been performed, suggesting more research is needed to determine the extent of efficacy of kanuka.

Manuka Honey

Manuka honey is honey that bees have produced using the flowers of the manuka tree (*Leptospermum scoparium*), a tree found in New Zealand and Australia [4]. While most types of honey exhibit antimicrobial effects through enzymatic production of hydrogen peroxide, manuka honey, also known as non-hydrogen peroxide honey, is unique in that it blocks bacterial growth through the enzyme methylglyoxal [3, 4, 13]. In fact, manuka honey has been found to have up to 100 times more of this enzyme than other honeys, and this may explain its superior antimicrobial effects over kanuka honey. However, large, randomized studies demonstrating the efficacy of manuka honey as a treatment for both acne and rosacea are lacking. Based on what we know regarding their mechanism of action and the pathophysiology behind acne and rosacea, we can hypothesize that manuka honey may be a better agent for acne, while kanuka honey may be a better agent for rosacea. However, compelling evidence for these different uses does not exist to date.

As the global health crisis of antibiotic resistance continues to grow, it is possible that the role of manuka honey in the treatment of acne and rosacea may become more prominent. Although resistance rates of antibiotics are rising, microbial resistance to honey has never been reported [13]. In addition to fighting acne and rosacea, we may soon be employing this natural agent in the fight against global health security.

Emerging Trends in Honey

As more research is being conducted on honey's effect on the skin, new formulations of honey-based cosmetics are being created. One such formulation includes cannabinoid

(CBD)-infused manuka honey. Cannabidiol has previously been studied for its sebostatic and anti-inflammatory effects on human sebocytes as a potential therapeutic agent for the treatment of acne [14]. CBD, derived from hemp, is non-psychoactive, has been shown to have calming and anti-inflammatory effects, and, when combined with the healing properties of manuka honey, may provide significant benefits for the skin. While much remains to be studied regarding the effectiveness of these agents, it will be interesting to see what role, if any, these products may have in the future of skin care.

Propolis

Propolis, also known as bee glue, is a resin-like product that is used by bees to close openings in their hives. Bees produce this substance by taking materials from plant parts, such as leaves and bark, and combining it with bee saliva, wax, and pollen to form a hard, waxlike product that when warm becomes soft and sticky [15]. Medicinal use of this product dates back as far as the ancient Greeks, Romans, and Egyptians, who noted propolis to be useful in the process of wound healing [1]. Propolis has since been proposed to have antimicrobial, antiviral, antifungal, anti-inflammatory, and anti-oxidant properties, making it useful in the treatment of various skin diseases.

Propolis in Acne

Clinical use of topical propolis extract has been studied as a potentially safe and cheap therapeutic option for management of facial acne. Propolis has been found to have greater efficacy against inflammatory acne lesions than noninflammatory ones, perhaps due to its anti-inflammatory properties [14]. Propolis has also been associated with a significant decrease in bacterial growth and colonization of acneiform lesions by *Cutibacterium acnes* (formerly *Propionibacterium acnes*) and *Staph epidermidis*, a result attributed to propolis' antibacterial properties [16]. In fact, in one study, propolis was found to be more effective than a topical antibiotic cream in reducing the severity/number of acne lesions. When a mixture of 20% propolis tree extract, 3% tree tea oil, and 10% aloe vera leaf juice (PTAC) was compared to 3% erythromycin cream, PTAC showed greater improvement and early action in reducing erythema of existing papules and scar inflammation from prior lesions [17]. This may in part be due to propolis having potential in increasing rates of wound healing [18]. Of note, the combination of all three ingredients in PTAC may exhibit a synergistic effect, as when each individual component is used alone, even in higher concentrations, a smaller effect is seen in reduction of number of acne lesions. However, propolis alone has shown reduction in seborrhea and greasiness of the skin, leading to overall improvement in skin appearance [16].

There is some controversy surrounding the tolerability of propolis in both topical and oral preparation. Propolis is generally thought to be well tolerated, due to the natural presence of wax and essential oils. Reported adverse effects associated with its use in acne patients include mild irritation and erythema, with the majority of users expressing good tolerability and no/minor post-therapy complaints [16].

However, propolis has a long history of association with occupational contact allergy, with the first published case dating back to 1915 in a beekeeper, and an increasing number of cases of allergic contact dermatitis being reported since the 1970s [15]. Higher frequencies have been most prominently observed in mid- and eastern European countries, where the extensive use of propolis for medical purposes is well-known, but rates have doubled in the United States as well, up from less than 2% to now 4.9% [15]. This increase is thought to be due to the growing trend of utilizing natural products, which are often thought by consumers to be safe and harmless but, in reality, are often unregulated and understudied for both their efficacy and their potential adverse effects.

The specific composition of propolis is highly variable, due to the regional variability of plant species in an area, making geographic region a major determinant of the final product [15, 19]. With over 180 different ingredients, and ingredients varying based on the region of production of propolis, it becomes very difficult to specify allergens in propolis, although many components have demonstrated strong sensitizing potential [19]. Today, most published cases of allergy are caused by the topical use of propolis for medicinal purposes, with cosmetic uses comprising a minority of cases [15]. Nonetheless, associated cases including propolis-containing cosmetic ointments, creams, facial lotions, and lip balms have demonstrated reactions ranging from severe cheilitis, perioral dermatitis, and generalized skin eruptions to appearance of patchy, eczematous lesions, proving propolis to not be as benign as once thought [15].

Propolis in Rosacea

To date, propolis has not been studied in rosacea, possibly due to these reported cases of allergic contact dermatitis. Patients with rosacea often have increased sensitivity of skin, and with the sensitizing potential of propolis, it may not be a viable treatment option for this population. However, anti-inflammatory mediators play a role in controlling the clinical signs and symptoms of rosacea, leading one to hypothesize that propolis could also be an effective agent. As more studies are conducted on propolis, it will be interesting to see where the future of this product in skincare will go.

Bee Venom

If you've ever been stung by a bee, chances are you've been injected with bee venom. Surprisingly, bee venom, the very toxin that makes these stings painful, has been used for many centuries as a therapeutic option in treating chronic inflammatory conditions [20].

This agent is particularly prominent in China and Eastern Europe and is becoming increasingly popular in Western countries. Traditional uses included musculoskeletal and rheumatological diseases such as sciatica, rheumatoid arthritis, multiple sclerosis, and low back pain [20]. Fortunately for us, this therapy has evolved from live bee stings and injectable venom to extracted and purified bee venom that can then be added to various topical agents. This evolution, in combination with the influence of the media, has helped pave the way for bee venom in the field of dermatology.

Purified bee venom (PBV) is natural bee venom that has been collected, diluted, and centrifuged in a laboratory to separate out contaminants, leaving behind a combination of active enzymes, peptides, and amino acids. Melitten, the major component of bee venom, suppresses inflammation through its inhibition of the enzyme phospholipase, which is found to be abundantly released in inflammatory conditions and acts to degrade various tissues and organs [20]. This anti-inflammatory effect has been the driving force behind bee venom's application in acne and rosacea.

Bee Venom in Acne

Although data is limited regarding bee venom's uses in acne, a few studies have found this product to have a significant therapeutic effect. PBV has been found to have antimicrobial properties against *Cutibacterium acnes* both in vitro and in vivo, making it a reasonable treatment modality to fight acne. One prospective study of subjects with mild to moderate acne evaluated improvement in clinical lesions following twice-daily application of PBV serum to the face. Following the 6-week study period, 77% of subjects showed improvement in the number and appearance of acne lesions when compared to baseline ($P < 0.001$), with the mean percentage improvement of lesion grade being 52.3% [21]. Statistically significant improvement was also seen in number of open and closed comedones ($P < 0.001$) as well as papules ($P < 0.05$), but not in pustules and nodules [21]. Importantly, none of the participants experienced any irritation or serious side effects, suggesting PBV to be a possible long-term option for the management of acne. This becomes especially noteworthy when comparing PBV to current dermatologist-recommended and FDA-approved acne products. Topical agents such as benzoyl peroxide, retinoids, and antibiotics (all level A recommendations) and salicylic acid (level B recommendation) are commonly used prescription and/or over-the-counter products that are recommended for once- to twice-daily application. (Of note, clinical recommendations can be categorized as level A, in which the recommendations are based on consistent and good-quality patient-oriented evidence, and level B, in which the recommendations are based on inconsistent or limited-quality patient-oriented evidence [22].) Yet, despite their proven efficacy, these agents have frequent reports of dryness, irritation, redness, itching, sun sensitivity, and peeling [22]. Such side effects are often limiting for patients, especially those with sensitive skin, and can create problems of treatment adherence. With the growing concerns of antibiotic resistance and the near negligible adverse effects associated with PBV, it may be time to introduce another player into the game.

The buzz surrounding bee venom doesn't just stop with acne. With the help of Hollywood pop culture and features in top beauty magazines, bee venom is breaking into the cosmetic industry. Consumers can now walk the aisles of their favorite beauty or department store and spot new lines of cosmetic brands selling bee venom face masks, creams, and cleansing balms that promise clearer, brighter skin. Although there is questionable validity to bee venom's efficacy on the skin, there may be some truth behind these statements. A study by Han et al., which sought to evaluate the effects of cosmetics containing PBV on acne, found that subjects using PBV products had significantly fewer inflammatory and non-inflammatory lesions than the control group ($P < 0.05$) [23]. An earlier in vitro study by Han et al. also showed PBV to have possible skin photo-protective effects through reduction of protein levels of matrix metalloproteinases, which are main contributors to the photo-aging process [24]. This “antiaging” effect of PBV was later studied in a clinical trial in healthy South Korean women, in which subjects were instructed to apply a 0.006% PBV-formulated facial serum twice daily for 12 weeks. A clinical improvement in facial wrinkles was found, with PBV serum treatment decreasing total wrinkle area, total wrinkle count, and average wrinkle depth [25]. Because extrinsic photodamage can lead to undesirable facial wrinkles, PBV may have beneficial effects against the intrinsic aging process of our skin, with headlines going as far as to call it “the natural alternative to botox” [26]. In fact, some dermatologists advocate that PBV results may mimic the effects of botulinum toxin, including increased circulation, tighter skin, and a temporary relaxation of facial muscle, motivating high-end vendors to place a pretty price tag of up to $42,000/ounce on nature’s product [18].

Bee Venom in Rosacea

Clinical studies regarding the use of bee venom in rosacea appear to be even more limited than those in acne. The New Zealand Ministry of Science and Innovation has proposed that a combination of manuka honey and PBV may reduce dark age spots and increase skin cell renewal, helping create stronger, healthier skin that may be less likely to have inflammatory flares, even if prone to rosacea [27]. Additionally, PBV may be an effective alternative treatment option for rosacea patients who struggle with acne, as many acne-fighting agents contain ingredients like benzyl peroxide that can aggravate rosacea. However, much more data must be compiled to understand the true effects, if any, PBV may have on rosacea.

Conclusion

The use of bee products continues to be studied in the field of complementary and alternative medicine. A definitive role for honey, propolis, and bee venom in the treatment of acne and rosacea cannot yet be established, due to the need for additional evidence and larger, randomized controlled trials with direct comparisons of these agents against standard treatments. Their versatile properties, however, do make these naturally derived agents a good potential option for those who have failed traditional treatment modalities, as well as those who are looking to avoid prescription medications and the harsh side effects that often accompany synthetic products. Bee products may also offer secondary benefits of improved skin texture, appearance, and healing abilities, leading to their increasing popularity in the skin care industry. As antimicrobial resistance continues to threaten global health security and more and more patients turn toward holistic treatment approaches, it may be wise to keep these agents in our back pocket.

References

1. Pasupuleti VR, Sammugam L, Ramesh N, Gan SH. Honey, propolis, and royal jelly: a comprehensive review of their biological actions and health benefits. Oxidative Med Cell Longev. 2017;2017:1259510.
2. Burlando B, Cornara L. Honey in dermatology and skin care: a review. J Cosmet Dermatol. 2013;12(4):306–13.
3. Molan P, Rhodes T. Honey: a biologic wound dressing. Wounds. 2015;27(6):141–51.
4. Avni. Honey for acne–use honey to remove acne and its scars. [online]. Available at: https://www.rapidhomeremedies.com/honey-for-acne.html.
5. Lu J, Carter DA, Turnbull L, Rosendale D, Hedderley D, Stephens J, et al. The effect of New Zealand kanuka, manuka and clover honeys on bacterial growth dynamics and cellular morphology varies according to the species. PLoS One. 2013;8(2):e55898.
6. Tomblin V, Ferguson LR, Han DY, Murray P, Schlothauer R. Potential pathway of anti-inflammatory effect by New Zealand honeys. Int J Gen Med. 2014;7:149–58.
7. Gannabathula S, Skinner MA, Rosendale D, Greenwood JM, Mutukumira AN, Steinhorn G, et al. Arabinogalactan proteins

contribute to the immunostimulatory properties of New Zealand honeys. Immunopharmacol Immunotoxicol. 2012;34(4):598–607.
8. Holt S. A New Zealand topical kanuka honey product can treat rosacea and reduce antibiotic resistance. Adv Integr Med. 2015;2(3):141–2.
9. Semprini A, Braithwaite I, Corin A, Sheahan D, Tofield C, Helm C, et al. Randomised controlled trial of topical kanuka honey for the treatment of acne. BMJ Open. 2016;6(2):e009448.
10. Braithwaite I, Hunt A, Riley J, Fingleton J, Kocks J, Corin A, et al. Randomised controlled trial of topical kanuka honey for the treatment of rosacea. BMJ Open. 2015;5(6):e007651.
11. van Zuuren EJ, Graber MA, Hollis S, Chaudhry M, Gupta AK, Gover M. Interventions for rosacea. Cochrane Database Syst Rev. 2005;20(3):CD003262.
12. Fingleton J, Sheahan D, Cave N, Brinded A, Weatherall M, Perrin K, et al. Topical kanuka honey for the treatment of rosacea. Focus Alternat Complement Ther. 2013;18(4):221–2.
13. Mandal MD, Mandal S. Honey: its medicinal property and antibacterial activity. Asian Pac J Trop Biomed. 2011;1(2):154–60.
14. Olah A, Toth BI, Borbiro I, Sugawara K, Szollosi AG, Czifra G, et al. Cannabidiol exerts sebostatic and antiinflammatory effects on human sebocytes. J Clin Invest. 2014;124(9):3713–24.
15. de Groot AC. Propolis: a review of properties, applications, chemical composition, contact allergy, and other adverse effects. Dermatitis. 2013;24(6):263–82.
16. Mohammad Ali BM, Ghoname NF, Hodeib AA, Elbadawy MA. Significance of topical propolis in the treatment of facial acne vulgaris. Egypt J Dermatol Venerol. 2015;35:29–36.
17. Mazzarello V, Donadu MG, Ferrari M, Piga G, Usai D, Zanetti S, et al. Treatment of acne with a combination of propolis, tea tree oil, and Aloe vera compared to erythromycin cream: two double-blind investigations. Clin Pharmacol. 2018;10:175–81.
18. Toreti VC, Sato HH, Pastore GM, Park YK. Recent progress of propolis for its biological and chemical compositions and its botanical origin. Evid Based Complement Alternat Med. 2013;2013:697390.
19. Freedman J, Griggs J, De Padova MP, Tosti A. What's the "buzz" about propolis? Propolis-induced systemic contact dermatitis. Contact Dermatitis. 2019;80(1):65–7.
20. Ali M. Studies on bee venom and its medical uses. Int J Adv Res Technol. 2012;1(2):69–83.

21. Han SM, Pak SC, Nicholls YM, Macfarlane N. Evaluation of anti-acne property of purified bee venom serum in humans. J Cosmet Dermatol. 2016;15(4):324–9.
22. Zaenglein AL, Pathy AL, Schlosser BJ, Alikhan A, Baldwin HE, Berson DS, et al. Guidelines of care for the management of acne vulgaris. J Am Acad Dermatol. 2016;74(5):945–73.
23. Han SM, Lee KG, Pak SC. Effects of cosmetics containing purified honeybee (Apis mellifera L.) venom on acne vulgaris. J Integr Med. 2013;11(5):320–6.
24. Han S, Lee K, Yeo J, Kweon H, Woo S, Lee M, et al. Inhibitory effect of bee venom against ultraviolet B induced MMP-11 and MMP-3 in human dermal fibroblasts. J Apic Res. 2007;46(2):94–8.
25. Han SM, Hong IP, Woo SO, Chun SN, Park KK, Nicholls YM, et al. The beneficial effects of honeybee-venom serum on facial wrinkles in humans. Clin Interv Aging. 2015;10:1587–92.
26. New You website. Editorial: the price of beauty – Bee-Tox. [online]. Available at: https://www.newyou.com/beauty/price-beauty/.
27. BeeBio website. Clinically proven results. [online]. Available at: https://beebioskin.com/pages/clinically-proven-results.

Chapter 7
Dietary Modifications for Acne and Rosacea

Jacquelyn Dosal and Marissa Ceresnie

Abbreviation

DAO Diamine oxidase

Dietary Modifications for Acne

Affecting up to 50 million Americans each year, acne is the most common skin condition in the United States [1]. However, observations of non-Westernized societies of Inuit, Okinawa, and Kitavan in Papua New Guinea and Aché in Paraguay show no evidence of acne [2–4]. Interestingly, after assimilation into Western society, the prevalence of acne grew to match that of civilized society in the Inuit and decedents of rural African populations in Kenya, Zambia, and Bantu in South Africa [5–7]. Research

J. Dosal (✉)
Department of Dermatology, Skin Associates of South Florida, Coral Gables, FL, USA

M. Ceresnie
Nova Southeastern University College of Osteopathic Medicine, Davie, FL, USA

R. N. Rupani, P. A. Lio (eds.), *Integrative Dermatology*,
https://doi.org/10.1007/978-3-030-58954-7_7

suggests this discrepancy is not a coincidence, and may be attributable to diet and genetics, as foods consumed by these isolated communities have substantially different characteristics, such as a much lower glycemic index, than the Western diet, which consists largely of refined carbohydrates, dairy products, red meat, and free fatty acids [4, 8].

Although the role of diet and acne has been controversial in the past century among medical professionals, the vast majority of acne patients believe diet can affect acne. In a 2016 survey, most participants thought fried, greasy foods caused acne, followed by chocolate, dairy, soda, caffeine, refined carbohydrates, and sugar [9]. Recently, the IL-1A (-889C/T) gene polymorphism was found to be associated with diet as a risk factor for acne, suggesting individuals may be genetically predisposed to have acne that is exacerbated by certain foods [10]. While reliable clinical data is limited on specific foods causing breakouts, the American Academy of Dermatology suggests that patients be encouraged to pay attention to foods or beverages that worsen their acne and observe the effect of abstaining from that particular product [11].

It is hypothesized that the branched chain amino acids, such as leucine, and glucose from foods in the Western diet increase sebogenesis, keratinocyte proliferation, lipogenesis, and inflammation, creating an optimal environment for acne development and *Cutibacterium acnes (C. acnes)* overgrowth. This is done through stimulation of the androgen receptor, which is activated by downregulation of FOXO1 transcription factor and upregulation of mTOR1 transcription factor by hyperinsulinemia and IGF-1 [12]. FOXO1 suppression has also been shown in vitro to increase human primary T cells, a key initiator of inflammation, independently from the toll-like receptor 2/4-mediated follicular inflammation induced by *C. acnes*, and studies have confirmed sebaceous gland inflammation alone is sufficient to develop acne (Fig. 7.1) [16, 17].

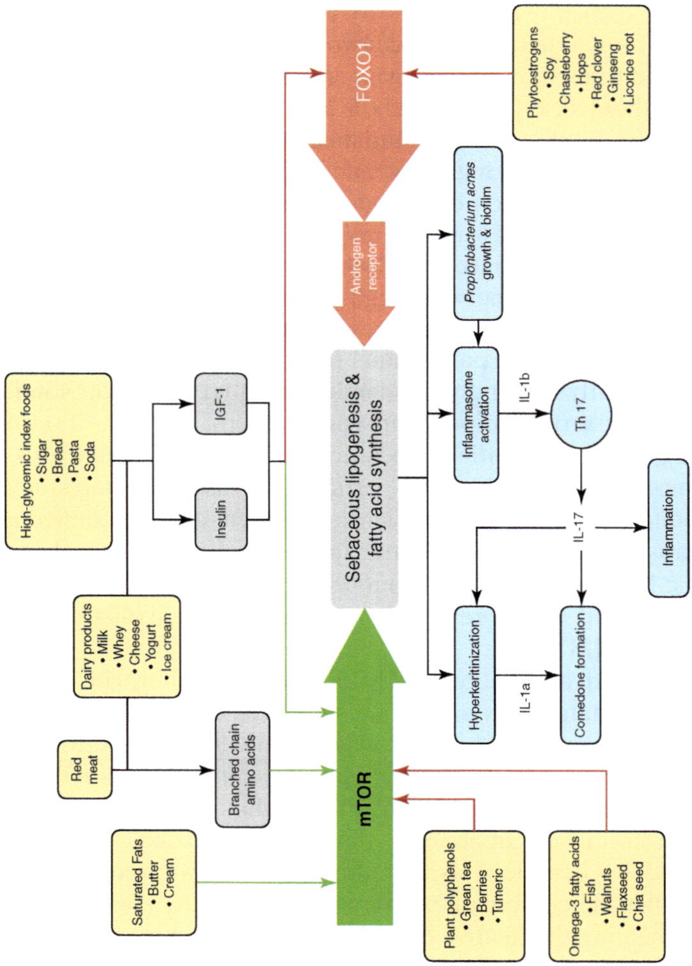

Figure 7.1 Proposed mechanisms of food groups studied to exacerbate acne development [12–15]

Low-Glycemic Index and Low-Glycemic Load Diet

Glycemic load is based on the rate sugar is released into the blood, which is determined by the ratio of carbohydrate to fiber present in a given food. Two individual randomized controlled trials showed improvement of acne on a low-glycemic load diet [18, 19]. Conversely, a 2015 Cochrane review of the two trials showed no statistically significant difference between low- and high-glycemic load diets on reducing non-inflammatory lesion counts at 12 weeks among the total 75 participants [11]. However, multiple additional studies have been conducted since the Cochrane review publication that supports the link between high-glycemic foods and acne.

Following the Cochrane review in 2016, a cross-sectional study involving 86 participants found patients with acne had significantly higher glycemic index and glycemic load, as well as lower serum adiponectin compared to the control, also suggesting a potential association of acne and insulin resistance [20]. In 2017, a 64-participant cross-sectional study found individuals with moderate to severe acne consumed a statistically significant greater total carbohydrate and glycemic load and displayed significantly higher levels of insulin, IGF-1, and insulin resistance compared to individuals without acne [21].

Beyond associations, a 2016 study by Fabbrocini et al. showed statistically significant improvement in acne with a 6-month course of both a low-glycemic diet and metformin therapy in male patients with acne resistant to common treatments. The positive effect of this combination suggests that pharmaceutical treatments that modify insulin sensitivity could be beneficial as an adjunct to a low-glycemic diet, though the combination approach used in the study makes delineating the relative contribution of each impossible [22].

A ketogenic diet, classically characterized as very-low-carbohydrate diet with a proportional increase in protein and fat to induce a state of metabolic ketosis, has been proposed as potentially beneficial to reduce acne; however, no trials have been completed to provide evidence. Of note, a recent 2019 study found 50% of acne patients have severe protein deficiency, consuming <30 g/day [23]. This deficiency makes sense, as low-protein diets are often high in carbohydrates, and previous studies have shown the relation between acne and a hyperglycemic diet [17–20]. Protein deficiency also impairs cytokine production and cell-mediated immunity, which is essential in the body's defense system [24]. According to the literature, the ketogenic diet has been found to reduce several inflammatory markers and reduce insulin and blood glucose levels, interfering in the IGF-1 signaling cascade that leads to the development of acne. Caution is advised; however, a high-protein diet can potentially lead to renal damage, as seen in some animal studies [25].

Dairy Products

Despite their relatively low-glycemic index, milk products have been found to increase postprandial insulin levels three- to sixfold [26]. Milk contains many components promoting increased mTOR1 signaling that may ultimately lead to the development of acne: IGF-1, whey protein, glutamine, branched chain amino acids, saturated fats, and microRNA [27–31]. In addition, it has been reported that 75–90% of milk products in the United States come from pregnant cows, whose milk contains higher amounts of DHEA, androstenedione, and testosterone [32, 33]. Activation of the estrogen and androgen receptors by these hormones leads to increased microRNA-21, enhancing PI3K–AKT signaling and reducing the nuclear activity of FOXO1 transcription factor that is associated with sebaceous lipogenesis at suppressed levels [34, 35].

In 2018, a systematic review and meta-analysis of dairy intake and acne included 14 observational studies on individuals 7–30 years old (n = 78,529). It concluded that any dairy product, such as milk, yogurt, and cheese, was associated with an increased odds ratio for acne, regardless of the amount or frequency, compared to no intake. Among dairy products, yogurt and low-fat/skim milk both had the highest odds ratio overall, and cheese had a borderline high odds ratio [36]. The whey content of these products is recognized to be the most acnegenic component, as whey protein is often added to supplement the calories in skim and reduced fat milk [12]. Intake of one or more glasses of any milk a day was also associated with a higher odds ratio compared to two to six glasses per week and less than weekly [36].

Another 2018 meta-analysis confirmed the increased risk of moderate and severe acne with consumption of milk, especially skim milk, and high intake of milk. Geographically, a significant association was found in both America (OR = 1.16) and Europe (OR = 1.28), but not in Asia, Africa, or South America [37]. To further investigate this, Juhl et al. conducted a Mendelian randomization study investigating the relation between adult acne and milk intake in 20,416 Danish adults with the lactase persistence gene LCT-13910 C/T. Interestingly, this study did not find any observational or genetic association between milk intake and acne among their population of Danish adults. While these results are limited due to a low prevalence of lactase non-persistence (6%), this study suggests lactose intolerance among this population may have a stronger relation to acne development, since the meta-analysis did show a significant correlation with milk and acne among Europeans [38].

Whey protein, a popular supplement among bodybuilders and a by-product of milk during cheese production, is another proposed acne instigator. In a study of five males ages 19–35 by Simonart, all five developed acne after consuming whey protein concentrates, three of which had no prior history of acne [39]. Another study by Cengiz et al. in 2017 of six men aged 16–18 observed all six men developed acne only to the trunk after beginning whey protein supplementation [40]. Although sample sizes are small in each of these studies, it is noteworthy that all participants in both studies developed acne lesions after ingesting whey protein, and this suggests whey protein restriction could be helpful in reducing acne.

Mediterranean Diet

In 2012, Skroza et al. conducted the first and only study to date on the association between the Mediterranean diet and acne. It included 93 cases and 200 controls and found that a Mediterranean diet demonstrated a protective role in acne pathogenesis with a Mediterranean diet score > 6. Adherence to the Mediterranean diet was categorized into scores in this study, with 0–2 as low, 3–6 as moderate, and 7–9 as high adherence. The cutoff value of 6 had a 94% sensitivity and 20% specificity for the protective effect of the Mediterranean diet on acne [41].

The Mediterranean diet is characteristically composed of a high intake of minimally processed, seasonal, fresh, and locally grown plants, fruits, whole-grain products, potatoes, legumes, nuts, and seeds. Olive oil is the main source of fat, as there is a high ratio of monounsaturated to saturated fatty acids. There is a relatively low intake of saturated animal fats and red meats. Moderate fish consumption provides omega-3 fatty acids, along with nuts and seeds. Low to moderate amounts of dairy, mostly as cheese and yogurt, limit the amount of branched chain amino acids in the diet. Concentrated sugars or honey is ingested only a few times per week, and red wine is drunk with meals in low to moderate amounts [42]. Generally, the Mediterranean diet has a low-glycemic index, and there has been research showing its beneficial role on coagulation and inflammatory processes by decreasing the oxidative stress by providing a significant amount of antioxidant vitamins [41, 43, 44].

Plant-Based Diet

It has been hypothesized that plant-based foods and spices could improve acne vulgaris through a variety of mechanisms, with many of them possibly affecting more than one pathway. It is unclear if plant-based foods directly affect the human through insulin levels or act primarily through the gut microbiome. Plant foods high in fiber, such as those present in whole grains, vegetables, and fruit, slow digestion and slowly release sugar in carbohydrates into the blood stream, contributing to a lower glycemic load [45].

Plant-based sources of polyphenols, through an unknown mechanism, appear to improve insulin sensitivity. Examples of these foods include olive leaf, berries, grapes, red wine, cinnamon, and green tea. Berry extract was shown in vitro to reduce glucose uptake by human intestinal epithelial cells, and green tea extract reduced the quantity of acne lesions in postadolescent women in a randomized, double-blind controlled trial [45–47]. In addition, turmeric has been suggested to improve acne by stabilizing blood sugar and wielding antimicrobial and anti-inflammatory properties by suppressing reactive oxygen species produced by *C. acnes* and pro-inflammatory cytokines [48–50].

Phytoestrogens present in plants have shown to have activity similar to estrogen, which seems to lower androgens through negative feedback and decrease sebaceous gland size, sebum production, and acne [50]. Soy products are particularly high in the phytoestrogen isoflavone. Chasteberry fruit, hops, and red clover were also shown to bind estrogen receptors, and ginseng and licorice root show some estrogen activity without binding to the estrogen receptor [45, 51, 52].

Chocolate

Being rich in phenolic antioxidants such as flavonoids, chocolate is often touted for its positive health effects and even shown to be protective against cardiovascular disease and diabetes [53–55]. While studies from the 1960s and 1970s did not demonstrate an association between chocolate and acne, many recent studies have found a strong correlation between dark chocolate intake and acne outbreaks [56–60]. A recent study found dark chocolate to increase both epidermal corneocyte desquamation and gram-positive microorganisms present on the facial skin, potentially leading to acne. In search of an explanation, researchers have found that components of cocoa increase production of interleukin-1 beta (IL-1B) and *C. acnes*-induced IL-1B potentiation, leading to hypercornification of keratinocytes and eventual desquamation. It is also possible chocolate flavonoids act to exacerbate acne by modifying the gut microbiome, leading to conditions assisting in skin colonization by *C. acnes* [55].

Salt

Very little data is available on the role of excessive salt consumption and acne. A 2015 study showed 76% of patients with acne consumed amounts of sodium chloride higher than the recommended daily allowance compared to 46.7% of controls. The study also showed sodium consumption was highest in participants with a younger age of acne onset [61]. Further investigation is warranted to determine the part salty foods play in acne exacerbations.

Conclusion

Acne seems to be a disease exclusive to Westernized civilizations, and diet is suspected to play an integral role in its pathogenesis. Diets high in glycemic load, dairy, and chocolate have shown to exacerbate acne significantly in clinical trials, while Mediterranean diets and plant-based diets seem to play a protective role against acne development. Further research is warranted to examine clinical associations with larger population sizes and investigate acne-causing mechanisms behind specific foods. Genetic studies point to specific polymorphisms predisposing to diet-induced acne exacerbations, so it is important to encourage patients to be aware and keep track of specific foods that may trigger their acne breakouts.

Dietary Modifications for Rosacea

Dietary modifications for rosacea have long been recognized as a crucial tool in the treatment of rosacea, possibly even a prototype for dietary modifications in dermatology. Rosacea was first reported in the fourteenth century and immediately correlated with excessive alcohol consumption [62].

Foods and Drinks to Avoid in Rosacea

According to a survey from the National Rosacea Society, 78% of rosacea patients reported changing their diet to avoid rosacea exacerbations, and 95% of these patients noted improvement with a dietary change [63]. A plethora of foods and beverages were identified to trigger rosacea; Table 7.1 includes information based on a survey by the National Rosacea Society [64].

Trying to understand why certain foods flare rosacea is complex and diverse. Food sensitivities in one rosacea patient may be completely different from another rosacea patient. There are several categories of foods and drinks that can be avoided and should be systematically evaluated. Avoidance of triggers is very important in rosacea, whether dietary or not. It not only helps repress active disease, but it also slows down the progression of this chronic disease, which does not currently have a cure.

Foods That May Flare Rosacea

1. Alcohol
2. Heat-related foods—hot coffee, tea, soups, hot chocolate, etc.
3. Spicy foods (capsaicin-related)
4. Histamine-containing foods, or histamine promoters
5. Niacin-containing foods
6. Cinnamaldehyde-related foods
7. Generally unhealthy foods that promote inflammation and hormone imbalance, including processed foods and sugary foods

Table 7.1 Comprehensive list of foods reported to trigger rosacea

Beverages	Alcohol, tea, coffee, hot chocolate, hot cider, kombucha, energy drinks, milk, kefir, soda, cold drinks
Dairy	Yogurt, sour cream, cheese, kefir, buttermilk, milk
Flavorings/spices/condiments	Spicy foods, vanilla, soy sauce, yeast extract, vinegar, cayenne pepper, red pepper, chili pepper, mustard, horseradish, cinnamon, cloves, cumin, fenugreek, ginger, apple cider vinegar, mayonnaise, ketchup
Fruits	Avocado, citrus, banana, plum, raisin, figs, dried fruits, papaya, pineapple, strawberries
Vegetables	Eggplant, spinach, tomato, sauerkraut, green peas, potatoes, dried shiitake mushrooms
Beans/legumes/nuts	Broad leaf beans (lima, navy, pea), legumes, peanuts, nuts
Pantry/processed foods	Sugar, sourdough bread, pickles, olives, wheat germ, food additives, brown rice, whole wheat, fortified and enriched foods, white flour, fried foods, vegetable oils, tofu, wet noodles
Meats/poultry/fish	Cured meats (bacon, sausage), canned/smoked fish, tuna, mackerel, salmon, sardines, mahi-mahi, egg whites, shellfish, liver, chicken breast, turkey, pork, ground beef, squid
Dessert	Chocolate, sugar

The use of a food diary is encouraged to avoid nutritional deficiencies and sweeping avoidance of food groups

1. *Alcohol*

Alcohol has been long noted to flare rosacea and has been demonstrated to accelerate the progression of rosacea [65]. The mechanism of action of alcohol-induced rosacea or flaring may involve several pathways. Alcohol vasodilates blood vessels, which can lead to flushing and cutaneous temperature elevation, resulting in local heat, which is a known trigger for rosacea. Alcohol also increases pro-inflammatory cytokines, and may induce cell cycle activators, which could contribute to epidermal hyperproliferation in rosacea [66–68]. Red wine, in particular, is well-known to flare rosacea, but exacerbations have also been reported with beer, champagne, and liquor [64].

2. *Hot Foods*

Thirty-three percent of survey respondents reported hot coffee as a trigger, while 30% reported hot tea as a trigger [63]. Both hot cider and hot cocoa have also been reported to trigger rosacea, as has chocolate on its own. In a randomized clinical trial, patients with current rosacea consumed caffeinated coffee and water at different temperatures. Neither water nor coffee at 22 °C leads to flushing, while both coffee and water at 60 °C lead to flushing with similar temporal nature and intensity, leading the author to conclude that heat, not caffeine, promotes flushing [69].

3. *Spicy Foods*

The common denominator in spicy foods that may be responsible for rosacea is capsaicin. Capsaicin is what gives a food its spice and heat and works via the transient receptor potential (TRP) vanilloid channels (TRPV1–6), which are located on keratinocytes and neural, endothelial, and immune cells. These receptors are activated by increased temperature and capsaicin, causing vasodilation and inflammation-induced hyperalgesia [70–72]. Capsaicin is an active component of chili peppers and can be found in hot pepper sauces and peppers, mainly cayenne, red, chili, jalapeno, peppercorn, black, and white varieties. Other spicy foods not containing capsaicin may also trigger rosacea symptoms, such as mustard, horseradish, cinnamon, cloves, cumin, fenugreek, and ginger.

4. *Histamine-Containing Foods*

It is estimated that 1% of the population is intolerant to histamine [73], which results from excessive histamine accumulation or insufficient breakdown [74]. This can result from low levels of diamine oxidase (DAO), which is the main enzyme responsible for breaking down histamine. Many of the foods known to trigger rosacea contain high amount of histamine or trigger its release. Of note, alcohol both contains high amounts of histamine and also directly releases histamine from mast cells. Furthermore, alcohol dehydrogenase inhibits DAO, leading to even more histamine accumulation [74]. McCusker and Sibdbury hypothesized that erythrotelangiectatic rosacea is more common in adults due to consumption of a more diverse palate of foods containing histamine and consumption of alcohol [74]. Patients with rosacea and histamine intolerance may benefit from a low-histamine diet and taking active measures to increase diamine oxidase. Supplemental DAO is available, as well as DOA cofactors such as vitamin C, copper, and pyridoxine (vitamin B6), which may help reduce the degradation of DAO in the setting of deficiency [73]. A low-histamine diet can be extremely restrictive and lead to nutritional deficiencies; therefore, it should only be employed if noticeable amelioration of rosacea symptoms is noted within 6 weeks of dietary modification. Taking an antihistamine about 2 h before a meal may also mitigate the effects of histamine [75].

Foods That Contain or Release Histamine

Histamine-Rich Foods to Avoid in Histamine-Sensitive Individuals

- Leftovers, aged, or fermented foods
- Fermented or sour dairy: cheese (especially aged), yogurt, sour cream, kefir, buttermilk
- Fermented foods: sauerkraut, vinegar, soy sauce, kefir, yogurt, kombucha, sourdough bread
- Fermented alcohol: wine, champagne, beer
- Vinegar-containing foods: apple cider vinegar, pickles, mayonnaise, olives, ketchup
- Cured meats: sausages, salami, bacon, pepperoni, lunch meats, hot dogs

- Dried fruits: raisins, prunes, figs, dates, apricots
- Fruits: citrus, avocado
- Nuts: walnuts, cashews, peanuts
- Vegetables: eggplant, spinach, tomatoes
- Canned or smoked fish and certain fish: sardines, tuna, mackerel, mahi-mahi, anchovies

Histamine-liberating foods: Alcohol, bananas, citrus, chocolate/cocoa, egg whites, legumes, milk, nuts, papaya, pineapple, shellfish, spices, strawberries, tomatoes, wheat germ, food additives (colors, preservatives, stabilizers, flavorings)

Diamine oxidase-blocking foods: alcohol, energy drinks, black tea, mate tea, green tea

5. *Niacin-Containing Foods*

Niacin is a commonly known cause of flushing. A seemingly discordant group of foods contains niacin: liver, yeast, avocadoes, spinach, chicken breast, tuna, turkey, salmon, anchovies, pork, ground beef (leaner varieties more than fattier varieties), peanuts, brown rice, whole wheat, mushrooms, green peas, potatoes, fortified and enriched foods, crustaceans, and dried shiitake mushrooms. Niacin-containing foods work on the G protein-coupled receptor 109A in dermal Langerhans cells, which increases the release of prostaglandins. This results in erythema, flushing, warmth, stinging, and itching [12]. Aspirin may reduce the effects of niacin-containing foods in those patients affected by them [75]. The flavonoid luteolin has also been used in animal studies to reduce niacin flush [76].

6. *Cinnamaldehyde-Containing Foods*

Cinnamaldehyde gives cinnamon its characteristic flavor. It is also found in tomatoes, citrus fruits, and chocolate. Cinnamaldehyde, in addition to mustard oil, activates the transient receptor potential ankyrin-1 (TRPA1) and may contribute to flushing [70, 77, 78].

New data may point to another group of triggers for rosacea similar to cinnamaldehyde-containing foods. Cold drinks and formalin-containing foods (fish, squid, tofu, wet noodles) increase substance P via TRPA1 channels on sensory neurons [12]. This secretes pro-inflammatory cytokines and neuropeptides. While cold drinks have not been traditionally associated with rosacea flares, cold weather has been implicated [79], despite both activating the TRPA1 receptor [71].

7. *Generally Unhealthy Foods*

This category includes sugary foods, white flour, starches, processed oils such as vegetable oils, hydrogenated oils, fried foods, processed meats, soda, energy drinks, preservatives, and additives. Processed foods spike insulin levels, contain pro-inflammatory oils, and wreak havoc on both the gut and the skin [12]. Focus should be on consuming freshly prepared whole foods, prepared freshly and not from a package.

The list of trigger foods for rosacea is long and diverse. Individual patients are likely to note variations and their own individual triggers. The authors do not recommend eliminating all of the listed foods. Instead, a food diary may help identify individual triggers and allow a varied diet, as not all categories of food will trigger rosacea in every patient.

Food and Drinks That May Improve Rosacea

Gut Health-Promoting Foods

Using the gut as a target intervention for rosacea is a novel and emerging area of therapeutics; however, the gut–brain–skin axis is not a new one [80]. Gut dysfunction/dysbiosis has been recognized to result in cutaneous manifestations; therefore, it is a plausible theory that dietary changes to support gut health may help improve symptoms in the skin by lowering inflammation caused by gut dysfunction/dysbiosis.

Rosacea has been linked with many conditions related to digestion, including *Helicobacter pylori* infection, small intestinal bacterial overgrowth (SIBO), celiac disease, irritable bowel disease, and even inflammatory bowel disease. Moreover, there are reports that the treatment of these conditions may result in improvement of rosacea symptoms [81–83]. Some rosacea patients with a degree of pancreatic insufficiency showed improvement of rosacea symptoms after treatment with pancreatic enzymes [84]. A case report by Kendall showed significant improvement of rosacea within 1 week of a high-fiber diet that reduced gut transit time to less than 30 h [85]. Since SIBO has been linked to decreased gut motility and rosacea, the postulated intervention of a high-fiber diet may also prove to be useful. Further, incorporating a plant-based fiber-rich diet also improves the composition of the gut microbiome in addition to improving gut motility time. Without fiber, mice studies show that pathogenic organisms proliferate rapidly in the gut and begin to digest the protective mucosal layer [86].

New data and hypotheses link the gut microbiome to rosacea [87]. The gut microbiome is very diverse and dynamic, impacted by many factors, including nutrition, supplements, stress, and medications. It has been postulated that gut dysbiosis actually can activate the plasma kallikrein–kinin pathways, leading to eventual neurogenic inflammation [87, 88]. A study with Korean women showed that compared to controls, patients with rosacea had an altered microbiome and an increase in *Acidaminococcus*, which alters gut barrier function by consumption of intestinal glutamate [89].

Both probiotics and prebiotics have shown modulatory effects on numerous inflammatory disorders [90]. Although research in rosacea is lacking, anecdotal reports are numerous, and there is a hypothetical and plausible mechanism of action for their effect [91]. Prebiotics are nondigestible, fiber-rich foods that feed the gut microbes, encouraging healthy organisms and diversity, while probiotics are foods or supplements that contain beneficial microbes. Probiotics help modulate inflammation and T-cell immune function (T-cell mediated), helping to counteract harmful bacteria [70]. Oral probiotics have also been shown to improve skin barrier function, a key dysfunctional component in the pathogenesis of rosacea [92]. Probiotics also produce lactic acid, antimicrobial peptides, and mucous, which have been shown to eradicate *Helicobacter pylori*, improving rosacea symptoms [74, 93]. Fermented foods are the main source of probiotics and include sauerkraut, kombucha, kimchi, yogurt, kefir, and miso. Of interest, probiotic-rich foods are also high in histamine and, as noted above, may actually trigger flares in some patients, so caution is recommended. This illustrates the complex and often conflicting information through which rosacea patients must sift.

Another concept that has been postulated to be associated with rosacea is leaky gut syndrome. Leaky gut syndrome is not a medically recognized condition, but is generally embraced in functional medicine practices. Leaky gut has been described as increased intestinal permeability, allowing microbes and waste products into the bloodstream, producing an immune and inflammatory response. Activated charcoal, which binds intestinal toxins, has been postulated to improve rosacea. While drinks with activated charcoal have come into the market with the "detoxifying" claim, there is no current evidence of that improving rosacea. Achlorhydria has also been noted in some rosacea patients, which may be due to urease production by *H. pylori*, and is also involved in SIBO. Naturopaths will sometimes use supplemental hydrochloride in these cases, with some reported success [74]. While there is no accepted approach to treating leaky gut syndrome, common practice consists of dietary avoidance of gluten, processed and simple carbohydrates (especially sugar), dairy, refined oils, alcohol, and other processed foods, with the addition of prebiotic–/probiotic-rich foods and whole minimally processed foods. This is consistent with many of the recommendations already outlined.

Anti-inflammatory Foods

Omega-3 fatty acids deserve special attention with rosacea. Many Western individuals have a large imbalance in the ratio of omega-6 to omega-3 fatty acids, mostly due to ubiquitous use of soybean and corn oil. The incorporation of omega-3 fatty acids, as well as limiting the consumption of processed foods to lower intake of omega-6 fatty acids, may help shift the metabolic pathway of these fatty acids from a pro-inflammatory to an anti-inflammatory pathway. While not specifically studied in cutaneous rosacea, a study has shown improvement in dry eyes in rosacea patients with the use of an omega-3 fatty acid supplement [94]. Omega-3-rich foods include salmon, mackerel, flax seed, cod liver oil, oysters, anchovies, chia seeds, and walnuts.

Zinc is a mineral that serves as a cofactor to numerous enzymatic reactions in the body. While there is conflicting data, it is plausible that foods rich in zinc may benefit rosacea [70, 95, 96]. Foods rich in zinc include oysters, red meat, shellfish, legumes, seeds, and nuts.

Food/Drinks That May Increase or Decrease the Risk of Developing Rosacea

The foods that trigger flares in existing patients may not be the same as foods that increase the risk of *developing* rosacea. Large studies have analyzed alcohol, coffee, tea, chocolate, fatty foods, dairy, spicy foods, smoking, and obesity. The largest studies showed an increased risk of rosacea in a dose-dependent relationship with alcohol consumption. One study found a higher risk of rosacea with consumption of white wine and liquor as opposed to red wine [68]. Only 2% of alcoholics were noted to have rosacea in one study [97, 98], while other studies showed only marginal association or no association [99–101]. Frequent consumption of fatty foods was noted to have a doubled risk of developing rosacea in a Chinese study [102]. There was also an increased risk of rosacea noted with chocolate [103], frequent tea consumption [102], and obesity [104]. Coffee (more than four cups a day) [103], dairy [102], and current smoking [99, 101, 105] were found to be protective against rosacea. Previous smoking was associated with rosacea [105, 106], and despite being a common trigger for existing patients, spicy foods were not associated [102].

Conclusion

The list of dietary triggers is long and diverse for rosacea, and rosacea patients may receive conflicting information. As dietary triggers often vary on the individual level, and the list of potential foods to avoid is long, a food diary is recommended to aid the patient in identifying personal causes of exacerbations. In general, a whole foods diet with focus on plants (other than those known to trigger rosacea), fiber, and minimally processed foods is recommended.

References

1. Bickers DR, Lim HW, Margolis D, Weinstock MA, Goodman C, Faulkner E, et al. The burden of skin diseases: 2004 a joint project of the American Academy of Dermatology Association and the Society for Investigative Dermatology. J Am Acad Dermatol. 2006;55(3):490–500.
2. Schaefer O. When the Eskimo comes to town. Nutr Today. 1971;6:8–16.
3. Steiner PE. Necropsies on Okinawans; anatomic and pathologic observations. Arch Pathol. 1946;42(4):359–80.
4. Cordain L, Lindeberg S, Hurtado M, Hill K, Eaton SB, Brand-Miller J. Acne vulgaris: a disease of Western civilization. Arch Dermatol. 2002;138(12):1584–90.
5. Verhagen AR, Koten JW, Chaddah VK, Patel RI. Skin diseases in Kenya. A clinical and histopathological study of 3,168 patients. Arch Dermatol. 1968;98(6):577–86.
6. Ratnam AV, Jayaraju K. Skin diseases in Zambia. Br J Dermatol. 1979;101(4):449–53.

7. Park RG. The age distribution of common skin disorders in the Bantu of Pretoria, Transvaal. Br J Dermatol. 1968;80(11):758–61.
8. Wolf R, Matz H, Orion E. Acne and diet. Clin Dermatol. 2004;22(5):387–93.
9. Nguyen QG, Markus R, Katta R. Diet and acne: an exploratory survey study of patient beliefs. Dermatol Pract Concept. 2016;6(2):21–7.
10. Ibrahim AA, Salem RM, El-Shimi OS, Baghdady SMA, Hussein S. IL1A (−889) gene polymorphism is associated with the effect of diet as a risk factor in acne vulgaris. J Cosmet Dermatol. 2019;18(1):333–6.
11. American Academy of Dermatology. Can the right diet get rid of acne? [Online] Available at: https://www.aad.org/public/diseases/acne-and-rosacea/can-the-right-diet-get-rid-of-acne
12. Maarouf M, Platto JF, Shi VY. The role of nutrition in inflammatory pilosebaceous disorders: implication of the skin-gut axis. Australas J Dermatol. 2019;60(2):e90–8.
13. Melnik BC. Linking diet to acne metabolomics, inflammation, and comedogenesis: an update. Clin Cosmet Investig Dermatol. 2015;8:371–88.
14. Melnik BC. Acne vulgaris: the metabolic syndrome of the pilosebaceous follicle. Clin Dermatol. 2018;36(1):29–40.
15. Claudel JP, Auffret N, Leccia MT, Poli F, Dreno B. Acne and nutrition: hypotheses, myths and facts. J Eur Acad Dermatol Venereol. 2018;32(10):1631–7.
16. Mirdamadi Y, Bommhardt U, Goihl A, Guttek K, Zouboulis CC, Quist S, et al. Insulin and insulin-like growth factor-1 can activate the phosphoinositide-3-kinase/Akt/FoxO1 pathway in T cells in vitro. Dermato-endocrinology. 2017;9(1):e1356518.
17. Mirdamadi Y, Thielitz A, Wiede A, Goihl A, Papakonstantinou E, Hartig R, et al. Insulin and insulin-like growth factor-1 can modulate the phosphoinositide-3-kinase/Akt/FoxO1 pathway in SZ95 sebocytes in vitro. Mol Cell Endocrinol. 2015;415:32–44.
18. Smith RN, Mann NJ, Braue A, Makelainen H, Varigos GA. The effect of a high-protein, low glycemic-load diet versus a conventional, high glycemic-load diet on biochemical parameters associated with acne vulgaris: a randomized, investigator-masked, controlled trial. J Am Acad Dermatol. 2007;57(2):247–56.
19. Kwon HH, Yoon JY, Hong JS, Jung JY, Park MS, Suh DH. Clinical and histological effect of a low glycaemic load diet in treatment of acne vulgaris in Korean patients: a randomized, controlled trial. Acta Derm Venereol. 2012;92(3):241–6.

20. Cerman AA, Aktas E, Altunay IK, Arici JE, Tulunay A, Ozturk FY. Dietary glycemic factors, insulin resistance, and adiponectin levels in acne vulgaris. J Am Acad Dermatol. 2016;75(1):155–62.
21. Burris J, Rietkerk W, Shikany JM, Woolf K. Differences in dietary glycemic load and hormones in New York City adults with no and moderate/severe acne. J Acad Nutr Diet. 2017;117(9):1375–83.
22. Fabbrocini G, Izzo R, Faggiano A, Del Prete M, Donnarumma M, Marasca C, et al. Low glycaemic diet and metformin therapy: a new approach in male subjects with acne resistant to common treatments. Clin Exp Dermatol. 2016;41(1):38–42.
23. Garg S, Sangwan A. Dietary protein deficit and deregulated autophagy: a new clinico-diagnostic perspective in pathogenesis of early aging, skin, and hair disorders. Indian Dermatol Online J. 2019;10(2):115–24.
24. Lesourd BM. Nutrition and immunity in the elderly: modification of immune responses with nutritional treatments. Am J Clin Nutr. 1997;66(2):478S–84S.
25. Paoli A, Grimaldi K, Toniolo L, Canato M, Bianco A, Fratter A. Nutrition and acne: therapeutic potential of ketogenic diets. Skin Pharmacol Physiol. 2012;25(3):111–7.
26. Ostman EM, Liljeberg Elmstahl HG, Bjorck IM. Inconsistency between glycemic and insulinemic responses to regular and fermented milk products. Am J Clin Nutr. 2001;74(1):96–100.
27. Melnik BC. The pathogenic role of persistent milk signaling in mTORC1- and milk-microRNA-driven type 2 diabetes mellitus. Curr Diabetes Rev. 2015;11(1):46–62.
28. Melnik BC, Schmitz G. Role of insulin, insulin-like growth factor-1, hyperglycaemic food and milk consumption in the pathogenesis of acne vulgaris. Exp Dermatol. 2009;18(10):833–41.
29. Yasuda M, Tanaka Y, Kume S, Morita Y, Chin-Kanasaki M, Araki H, et al. Fatty acids are novel nutrient factors to regulate mTORC1 lysosomal localization and apoptosis in podocytes. Biochim Biophys Acta. 2014;1842(7):1097–108.
30. Melnik BC, Kakulas F, Geddes DT, Hartmann PE, John SM, Carrera-Bastos P, et al. Milk miRNAs: simple nutrients or systemic functional regulators? Nutr Metab (Lond). 2016;13:42.
31. Clatici VG, Voicu C, Voaides C, Roseanu A, Icriverzi M, Jurcoane S. Diseases of civilization - cancer, diabetes, obesity and acne - the implication of milk, IGF-1 and mTORC1. Mædica (Buchar). 2018;13(4):273–81.
32. Danby FW. Acne and milk, the diet myth, and beyond. J Am Acad Dermatol. 2005;52(2):360–2.

33. Gaiani R, Chiesa F, Mattioli M, Nannetti G, Galeati G. Androstenedione and testosterone concentrations in plasma and milk of the cow throughout pregnancy. J Reprod Fertil. 1984;70(1):55–9.
34. Regal P, Cepeda A, Fente C. Development of an LC-MS/MS method to quantify sex hormones in bovine milk and influence of pregnancy in their levels. Food Addit Contam Part A Chem Anal Control Expo Risk Assess. 2012;29(5):770–9.
35. Teng Y, Litchfield LM, Ivanova MM, Prough RA, Clark BJ, Klinge CM. Dehydroepiandrosterone-induces miR-21 transcription in HepG2 cells through estrogen receptor beta and androgen receptor. Mol Cell Endocrinol. 2014;392(1–2):23–36.
36. Juhl CR, Bergholdt HKM, Miller IM, Jemec GBE, Kanters JK, Ellervik C. Dairy intake and acne vulgaris: a systematic review and meta-analysis of 78,529 children, adolescents, and young adults. Nutrients. 2018;10(8):1049.
37. Dai R, Hua W, Chen W, Xiong L, Li L. The effect of milk consumption on acne: a meta-analysis of observational studies. J Eur Acad Dermatol Venereol. 2018;32(12):2244–53.
38. Juhl CR, Bergholdt HKM, Miller IM, Jemec GBE, Kanters JK, Ellervik C. Lactase persistence, milk intake, and adult acne: a mendelian randomization study of 20,416 Danish adults. Nutrients. 2018;10(8):1041.
39. Simonart T. Acne and whey protein supplementation among bodybuilders. Dermatology. 2012;225(3):256–8.
40. Cengiz FP, Cevirgen Cemil B, Emiroglu N, Gulsel Bahali A, Onsun N. Acne located on the trunk, whey protein supplementation: is there any association? Health Promot Perspect. 2017;7(2):106–8.
41. Skroza N, Tolino E, Semyonov L, Proietti I, Bernardini N, Nicolucci F, et al. Mediterranean diet and familial dysmetabolism as factors influencing the development of acne. Scand J Public Health. 2012;40(5):466–74.
42. Willett WC, Sacks F, Trichopoulou A, Drescher G, Ferro-Luzzi A, Helsing E, et al. Mediterranean diet pyramid: a cultural model for healthy eating. Am J Clin Nutr. 1995;61(6 Suppl):1402S–6S.
43. Ryan M, McInerney D, Owens D, Collins P, Johnson A, Tomkin GH. Diabetes and the Mediterranean diet: a beneficial effect of oleic acid on insulin sensitivity, adipocyte glucose transport and endothelium-dependent vasoreactivity. QJM. 2000;93(2):85–91.
44. Ambring A, Friberg P, Axelsen M, Laffrenzen M, Taskinen MR, Basu S, et al. Effects of a Mediterranean-inspired diet on blood

lipids, vascular function and oxidative stress in healthy subjects. Clin Sci (Lond). 2004;106(5):519–25.
45. Clark AK, Haas KN, Sivamani RK. Edible plants and their influence on the gut microbiome and acne. Int J Mol Sci. 2017;18(5):1070.
46. Kim Y, Keogh JB, Clifton PM. Polyphenols and glycemic control. Nutrients. 2016;8(1):17.
47. Lu PH, Hsu CH. Does supplementation with green tea extract improve acne in post-adolescent women? A randomized, double-blind, and placebo-controlled clinical trial. Complement Ther Med. 2016;25:159–63.
48. Kim T, Davis J, Zhang AJ, He X, Mathews ST. Curcumin activates AMPK and suppresses gluconeogenic gene expression in hepatoma cells. Biochem Biophys Res Commun. 2009;388(2):377–82.
49. Ghosh S, Banerjee S, Sil PC. The beneficial role of curcumin on inflammation, diabetes and neurodegenerative disease: a recent update. Food Chem Toxicol. 2015;83:111–24.
50. Wickenberg J, Ingemansson SL, Hlebowicz J. Effects of Curcuma longa (turmeric) on postprandial plasma glucose and insulin in healthy subjects. Nutr J. 2010;9:43.
51. Stevens JF, Maier CS. The chemistry of gut microbial metabolism of polyphenols. Phytochem Rev. 2016;15(3):425–44.
52. Powers CN, Setzer WN. A molecular docking study of phytochemical estrogen mimics from dietary herbal supplements. In Silico Pharmacol. 2015;3:4.
53. Katz DL, Doughty K, Ali A. Cocoa and chocolate in human health and disease. Antioxid Redox Signal. 2011;15(10):2779–811.
54. Ellam S, Williamson G. Cocoa and human health. Annu Rev Nutr. 2013;33:105–28.
55. Strat KM, Rowley TJ, Smithson AT, Tessem JS, Hulver MW, Liu D, et al. Mechanisms by which cocoa flavanols improve metabolic syndrome and related disorders. J Nutr Biochem. 2016;35:1–21.
56. Bowe WP, Joshi SS, Shalita AR. Diet and acne. J Am Acad Dermatol. 2010;63(1):124–41.
57. Caperton C, Block S, Viera M, Keri J, Berman B. Double-blind, placebo-controlled study assessing the effect of chocolate consumption in subjects with a history of acne vulgaris. J Clin Aesthet Dermatol. 2014;7(5):19–23.
58. Delost GR, Delost ME, Lloyd J. The impact of chocolate consumption on acne vulgaris in college students: a randomized crossover study. J Am Acad Dermatol. 2016;75(1):220–2.

59. Vongraviopap S, Asawanonda P. Dark chocolate exacerbates acne. Int J Dermatol. 2016;55(5):587–91.
60. Wolkenstein P, Machovcova A, Szepietowski JC, Tennstedt D, Veraldi S, Delarue A. Acne prevalence and associations with lifestyle: a cross-sectional online survey of adolescents/young adults in 7 European countries. J Eur Acad Dermatol Venereol. 2018;32(2):298–306.
61. El Darouti MA, Zeid OA, Abdel Halim DM, Hegazy RA, Kadry D, Shehab DI, et al. Salty and spicy food; are they involved in the pathogenesis of acne vulgaris? A case controlled study. J Cosmet Dermatol. 2016;15(2):145–9.
62. de Bersaques J. Historical notes on rosacea. Eur J Dermatol. 1995;5:16–22.
63. Drake L. Hot sauce, wine and tomatoes cause flare-ups, survey finds, 2005. [Online] Available at: https://www.rosacea.org/rr/2005/fall/article_3.php. Accessed 13 Apr 2019.
64. National Rosacea Society. Factors that may trigger rosacea flare ups. [Online] Available at: https://www.rosacea.org/patients/rosacea-triggers/factors-that-may-trigger-rosacea-flare-ups. Accessed 13 Apr 2019.
65. Higgins E, du Vivier A. Alcohol intake and other skin disorders. Clin Dermatol. 1999;17:437–41.
66. Smith KE, Fenske NA. Cutaneous manifestations of alcohol abuse. J Am Acad Dermatol. 2000;43(1 Pt 1):1–16; quiz 16–8.
67. Farkas A, Kemeny L, Szell M, Dobozy A, Bata-Csorgo Z. Ethanol and acetone stimulate the proliferation of HaCaT keratinocytes: the possible role of alcohol in exacerbating psoriasis. Arch Dermatol Res. 2003;295(2):56–62.
68. Li S, Cho E, Drucker AM, Qureshi AA, Li WQ. Alcohol intake and risk of rosacea in US women. J Am Acad Dermatol. 2017;76:1061–7.
69. Wilkin JK. Oral thermal-induced flushing in erythematotelangiectatic rosacea. J Invest Dermatol. 1981;76(1):15–8.
70. Weiss E, Katta R. Diet and rosacea: the role of dietary change in the management of rosacea. Dermatol Pract Concept. 2017;7(4):31–8.
71. Aubdool AA, Brain SD. Neurovascular aspects of skin neurogenic inflammation. J Investig Dermatol Symp Proc. 2011;15(1):33–9.
72. Early S. Vanilloid and melastatin transient receptor potential channels in vascular smooth muscle. Microcirculation. 2010;17(4):237–49.

73. Maintz L, Novak N. Histamine and histamine intolerance. Am J Clin Nutr. 2007;85:1185–96.
74. McCusker M, Sibdbury R. Nutrition and skin: kids are not just little people. Clin Dermatol. 2016;34:698–709.
75. Jacknin J. Therapeutic diets for skin disorders. In: Norman RA, Shenefelt PD, Rupani RN, editors. Integrative dermatology. New York: Weil Integrative Medicine Library, Oxford Press; 2014.
76. Papaliodis D, Boucher W, Kempuraj D, Theoharides TC. The flavonoid luteolin inhibits niacin-induced flush. Br J Pharmacol. 2008;153(7):1382–7.
77. Campbell TM, Neems R, Moore J. Severe exacerbation of rosacea induced by cinnamon supplements. J Drugs Dermatol. 2008;7(6):8–10.
78. Pozsgai G, Bodkin JV, Graepel R, Bevan S, Andersson DA, Brain SD. Evidence for the pathophysiological relevance of TRPA1 receptors in the cardiovascular system in vivo. Cardiovasc Res. 2010;87(4):760–8.
79. National Rosacea Society. Rosacea triggers survey. [Online] Available at: https://www.rosacea.org/patients/rosacea-triggers-survey. Accessed 13 Apr 2019.
80. Arck P, Handijski B, Hagen E, Pincus M, Bruenahl C, Bienenstock J, et al. Is there a 'gut-brain-skin axis'? Exp Dermatol. 2010;19(5):401–5.
81. Egeberg A, Weinstock LB, Thyssen EP, Gislason GH, Thyssen JP. Rosacea and gastrointestinal disorders: a population-based cohort study. Br J Dermatol. 2017;176(1):100–6.
82. Parodi A, Paolino S, Greco A, Drago F, Mansi C, Rebora A, et al. Small intestinal bacterial overgrowth in rosacea: clinical effectiveness of its eradication. Clin Gastroenterol Hepatol. 2008;6:759–64.
83. Gravina A, Federico A, Ruocco E, Lo Schiavo A, Masarone M, Tuccillo C, et al. Helicobacter pylori infection but not small intestinal bacterial overgrowth may play a pathogenic role in rosacea. United European Gastroenterol J. 2015;3:17–24.
84. Barba A, Rosa B, Angelini G, Sapuppo A, Brocco G, Scuro LA, et al. Pancreatic exocrine function in rosacea. Dermatologica. 1982;165:601–6.
85. Kendall SN. Remission of rosacea induced by reduction of gut transit time. Clin Exp Dermatol. 2004;29(3):297–9.
86. Desai MS, Seekatz AM, Koropatkin NM, Kamada N, Hickey CA, Wolter M, et al. A dietary fiber-deprived gut microbiota

degrades the colonic mucus barrier and enhances pathogen susceptibility. Cell. 2016;167(5):1339–53.
87. Musthaq S, Mazuy A, Jakus J. The microbiome in dermatology. Clin Dermatol. 2018;36:390–8.
88. Two AM, Del Rosso JQ. Kallikrein 5-mediated inflammation in rosacea: clinically relevant correlations with acute and chronic manifestations in rosacea and how individual treatments may provide therapeutic benefit. J Clin Aesthet Dermatol. 2014;7:20–5.
89. Nam JH, Yun Y, Kim HS, Kim HN, Jung HJ, Chang Y, et al. Rosacea and its association with enteral microbiota in Korean females. Exp Dermatol. 2017;27:37–42.
90. Chang Y-S, Trivedi MK, Jha A, Lin Y-F, Dimaano L, Garcia-Romero MT. Synbiotics for prevention and treatment of atopic dermatitis. JAMA Pediatr. 2016;170(3):236.
91. Bowe WP. Probiotics in acne and rosacea. Cutis. 2013;92:6–7.
92. Gueniche A, Benyacoub J, Philippe D, Bastien P, Kusy N, Breton L, et al. Lactobacillus paracasei CNCM I-2116 (ST11) inhibits substance P-induced skin inflammation and accelerates skin barrier function recovery in vitro. Eur J Dermatol. 2010;20(6):731–7.
93. Zheng PX, Fang HY, Yang HB, Tien NY, Wang MC, Wu JJ. Lactobacillus pentosus strain LPS16 produces lactic acid, inhibiting multidrug-resistant Helicobacter pylori. J Microbiol Immunol Infect. 2016;49(2):168–74.
94. Bhargava R, Chandra M, Bansal U, Singh D, Ranjan S, Sharma S. A randomized controlled trial of omega 3 fatty acids in rosacea patients with dry eye symptoms. Curr Eye Res. 2016;41(10):1274–80.
95. Sharquie KE, Najim RA, Al-Salman HN. Oral zinc sulfate in the treatment of rosacea: a double-blind, placebo-controlled study. Int J Dermatol. 2006;45(7):857–61.
96. Bamford JTM, Gessert CE, Haller IV, Kruger K, Johnson BP. Randomized, double-blind trial of 220 mg zinc sulfate twice daily in the treatment of rosacea. Int J Dermatol. 2012;51(4):459–62.
97. Higgins EM, du Vivier AW. Cutaneous disease and alcohol misuse. Br Med Bull. 1994;50(1):85–98.
98. Rosset M, Oki G. Skin diseases in alcoholics. Q J Stud Alcohol. 1971;32:1017–24.
99. Alinia H, Tuchayi SM, Patel NU, Patel N, Awosika O, Bahrami N, et al. Rosacea triggers: alcohol and smoking. Dermatol Clin. 2018;36:123–6.

100. Abram K, Silm H, Maaroos HI, Oona M. Risk factors associated with rosacea. J Eur Acad Dermatol Venereol. 2010;24(5):565–71.
101. Spoendlin J, Voegel JJ, Jick SS, Meier CR. A study on the epidemiology of rosacea in the UK. Br J Dermatol. 2012;167(3):598–605.
102. Yuan X, Huang X, Wang B, Huang Y, Zhang YY, Tang Y, et al. Relationship between rosacea and dietary factors: a multicenter retrospective case-control survey. J Dermatol. 2019;46:219–25.
103. Li S, Chen ML, Drucker AM, Cho E, Geng H, Qureshi AA, Li WQ. Association of caffeine intake and caffeinated coffee consumption with risk of incident rosacea in women. JAMA Dermatol. 2018;154(12):1394–400.
104. Li S, Cho E, Drucker AM, Qureshi AA, Li WQ. Obesity and risk for incident rosacea in US women. J Am Acad Dermatol. 2017;77(6):1083–7.e5.
105. Li S, Cho E, Drucker AM, Qureshi AA, Li WQ. Cigarette smoking and risk of incident rosacea in women. Am J Epidemiol. 2017;186:38–45.
106. Kucukunal A, Altunay I, Arici JE, Cerman AA. Is the effect of smoking on rosacea still somewhat of a mystery. Cutan Ocul Toxicol. 2016;35(2):110–4.

Chapter 8
Mind–Body Therapies

Keira L. Barr, Carol Ann Soutor, and Jessica Maria May Franklin

Introduction

One-third of adults who have acne expressed feeling embarrassed or self-conscious because of their skin. Although rosacea is estimated to affect only 10% of the population [1], its impact should not be underestimated. The pathogenesis of both of these conditions is multifactorial. One of these factors is stress. Stress can be both an inciting or exacerbating factor of the condition and an outcome of the condition itself.

Psychological Impact of Acne and Rosacea

It is well established that both acne and rosacea have a physical impact, such as disfigurement and permanent scarring, yet

K. L. Barr (✉)
Resilient Health Institute, Gig Harbor, WA, USA
e-mail: hello@drkeirabarr.com

C. A. Soutor
Department of Dermatology, University of Minnesota Medical Center, Minneapolis, MN, USA

J. M. M. Franklin
Edward Via College of Osteopathic Medicine – Virginia Campus, Blacksburg, VA, USA

R. N. Rupani, P. A. Lio (eds.), *Integrative Dermatology*,
https://doi.org/10.1007/978-3-030-58954-7_8

the long-lasting psychosocial effects that can impact a patient's quality of life often do not receive equal attention. Anxiety, depression, social isolation, and suicidal ideation are common comorbidities of acne and rosacea that cannot be overlooked in the management of these patients. Research suggests that the impact on quality of life can be alleviated by mind–body therapies including biofeedback, meditation, and hypnosis, with resultant stress management, stress reduction [2], and improvement in the clinical manifestations of acne and rosacea.

As acne is such a common skin disorder affecting approximately 85% of 11- to 30-year-olds, it is important to consider all contributing pathogenic factors when managing these patients [2]. Research has shown that adolescent patients with severe acne had a prevalence of depression of 18–29% compared to 5–8% of the general adolescent population [3]. Studies have highlighted that the affected population has a lower self-image, self-esteem, and sense of self-worth, leading to feelings of isolation, loneliness, depression, anxiety, and a higher rate of patients with suicidal ideation [4–8].

Of note, the impact of acne on quality of life is reported to be equal to that reported by patients with other chronic diseases including diabetes, back pain, and epilepsy, regardless of the degree of acne severity [9–11]. Even in mild forms, acne can have a detrimental psychological impact on patients, due to how they perceive their skin to be evaluated by others, which contributes to a higher level of stress, anxiety, and depression [12, 13].

An important consideration is that if left untreated, acne lesions can persist into adulthood, and these psychosocial effects may also impact socioeconomic status. Studies have highlighted higher unemployment rates and lower social status for patients with acne compared to adults without [14, 15].

Similar to acne, the psychosocial impact of rosacea can be significant regardless of clinical severity. This may be attributed to the difficulty of concealing the facial localization of the condition. A survey conducted by the National Rosacea Society involving more than 400 rosacea subjects found that

75% expressed feelings of low self-esteem, 70% embarrassment, 69% frustration, and 56% stripped of their happiness. It is not surprising, then, that a study found that depression is common among rosacea patients, with approximately 32% experiencing some level of depression [16].

Not only does the presence of acne contribute to a feeling of stress, but both acne and rosacea have also been found to be more common in those who experience a higher intensity of stress from life events than those without such events. In many patients, rosacea can be worsened or triggered by factors that provoke flushing, such as emotions of shame or embarrassment. For example, a study found that patients' rosacea lesions were preceded by a traumatic emotional experience, including death of a loved one, divorce, severe family turmoil, or a major medical problem [17]. For adult female acne sufferers, job stress was found to be an additional factor that correlated with greater acne severity. Another study linking acne exacerbation with emotional factors reported an increase in acne lesion counts days after an interview during which anger was intentionally elicited. Both the emotional state of the patient and the level of stress can not only impact the onset and severity of the condition, but evidence is growing that uncontrolled stress can also impede the recovery process [17, 18].

The Brain–Skin Connection

The skin and the central nervous system (CNS), derived from the same embryological origin, both communicate through a common biochemical language that involves shared neuroendocrine hormones, neurotransmitters, cytokines, and their respective receptors [19]. Because of this relationship, the skin is an organ that is strongly reactive to psychiatric and psychological conditions, and this dynamic may be significant in the pathogenesis of several skin diseases, including acne and rosacea.

The brain and the nervous system influence the skin's immune cells through various chemical messengers and receptors, which respond to stress and exert its effect on the skin mainly through the hypothalamic–pituitary–adrenal (HPA) axis and the sympathetic adrenal medullary (SAM) axis. When these responses are activated, stress hormones such as corticotropin-releasing hormone (CRH), glucocorticoids, and epinephrine are released, which results in a host of immune and physiologic reactions that can trigger or exacerbate skin conditions like acne and rosacea, as illustrated in Fig. 8.1.

In response to emotional distress, the HPA axis activates corticotropin-releasing hormone (CRH). CRH functions as a central coordinator for behavioral and neuroendocrine responses to stress. CRH then activates adrenocorticotropic hormone (ACTH) secretion from the pituitary, which in turn triggers the production of adrenal cortisol and glucocorticoids [19].

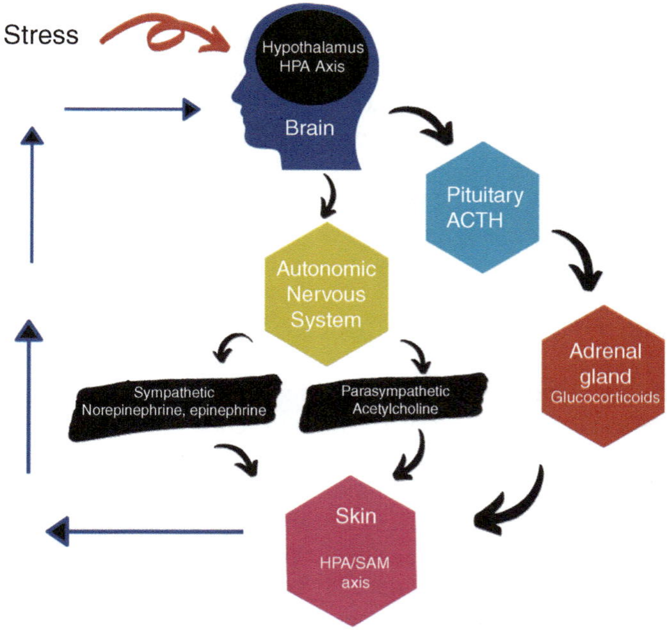

FIGURE 8.1 The central skin response and the skin peripheral stress response

Cortisol is the primary stress hormone that regulates a wide range of stress responses, and levels typically oscillate in response to the circadian rhythm; however, stress can significantly disrupt the cycle. Under stress conditions, cortisol levels are significantly upregulated, which can have a major impact on the immune system including secretion of cytokines and antibodies and a shift of the T helper (Th) 1 toward Th2 responses [20].

CRH also stimulates activation of the Sympathetic-Adrenal-Medullar (SAM) axis. An activated SAM triggers the adrenals to release catecholamines (norepinephrine and epinephrine), which alters blood flow, immune function, and the function of cells within the skin. This activation of the autonomic nervous system sets in motion the "fight, flight, or freeze" response associated with inflammation, in contrast to the parasympathetic response of "rest, repair, and digest" associated with relaxation and recovery.

Recent research highlights the skin both as an immediate stress perceiver and as a target of stress responses, because there are fully functional peripheral HPA and SAM systems within the skin [19]. This means that all of the stress hormones and their receptors are produced in skin cells, including epidermal and hair follicle keratinocytes, melanocytes, sebocytes, and mast cells, upon stress—reinforcing the bidirectional communication between the nervous, immune, and cutaneous systems [20].

Impact of Stress on Acne and Rosacea

Various mechanisms have been proposed for why stress may potentially aggravate acne vulgaris and rosacea. Researchers found that the release of adrenal androgens and glucocorticoids stimulated by CRH induces sebaceous hyperplasia, increases sebaceous lipogenesis, and upregulates sebocyte conversion of androgen precursors to testosterone. These activated sebocytes release cytokines, including IL1-alpha, IL-6, IL-11, TNF-alpha, INF-gamma, and PPAR-gamma, producing inflammation. There is also research suggesting that

Cutibacterium acnes itself can produce CRH through direct contact with keratinocytes, affecting infundibular keratinocyte differentiation [21–24]. Investigators have also found that substance P, a neuropeptide elicited from peripheral nerves by stress, can stimulate the proliferation of sebaceous glands and upregulate lipid synthesis in sebaceous cells, and trigger the release of pro-inflammatory cytokines from sebocytes, including IL-1, IL-6, and TNF-alpha. In addition, psychological stress can slow wound healing by up to 40%, which may be a factor in slowing the repair of acne lesions [25].

In rosacea, studies have highlighted that stress can trigger vasomotor reactions, resulting in vasodilation manifesting as blushing and facial redness typical of this condition. Vasodilatation can be produced by neuropeptides, cytokines, and vasoactive peptides upon stimulation by the SAM [20].

Although to date there has been a paucity of reported cases specifically addressing the role of stress management in acne and rosacea, the literature supports the role of mind–body techniques for managing, reducing, and alleviating stress and anxiety in individuals on the whole. It is from this perspective that we draw upon the evidence for consideration of using these techniques as an adjunct to managing these skin conditions.

Effects of Mind–Body Therapies on Acne and Rosacea

Mind-body therapies (MBTs) are a collection of practices and treatments that promote health and well-being utilizing the bidirectional relationship between the mind–brain–body. Commonly used MBTs include:

- *Meditation techniques*: Mindfulness including mindfulness-based stress reduction (MBSR), relaxation response, guided imagery, and autogenic training
- *Psychological approaches*: Biofeedback, cognitive behavioral therapy, and emotional freedom technique (EFT), and hypnotherapy
- *Breath work*: Pranayama yoga and other breathing techniques

- *Movement*: Yoga, Qi Gong, and Tai Chi
- *Body work*: Acupuncture, Reiki, and massage
- *Community and connection*: Support groups and spirituality
- *Creative therapy*: Music, writing, and art

Mind–body therapies (MBT) offer an array of benefits to the physical, psychological, and spiritual needs of our patients. Most of these therapies have their origins in ancient traditional healing practices. In the past 30 years, many of these therapies have become standardized and have evidence-based support for their efficacy in several physical and mental disorders [26–28]. In addition, there is evidence for their cost-effectiveness [29].

Table 8.1 summarizes some of the reported benefits of MBT. MBTs' modulation of the stress response is one of the

Table 8.1 Reported benefits of mind–body therapies

Role of stress in acne and rosacea	**Mind–body therapies' effects on acne and rosacea**
Psychosocial stress can trigger or exacerbate acne and rosacea	Downregulate the stress response
Patient's response to their acne and rosacea can create additional stress	Reduce inflammation, decrease sebum production
Stress can trigger inflammation, which is a key component in the pathogenesis of acne and rosacea	Activate the repair mechanisms of the skin to support allostasis
Stress can affect the barrier function of the skin	Reduce patients' manipulation of skin lesions
	Mitigate the psychological comorbidities, including anxiety, depression, and stigma
	Improve other quality-of-life measures
	Considered to be safe and cost-effective

main factors in their efficacy. The stress response is not necessarily just triggered by exposure to a specific stressor. The emotional response to the stressor plays a large part in the initiation of the stress response [30]. However, genetics, living conditions, resiliency, gender, and age are also factors in the stress response.

MBTs blunt the effect of a stressor by invoking the relaxation response, which stimulates the parasympathetic nervous system and downregulates the hypothalamus–pituitary–adrenocortical (HPA) axis and the sympathetic adrenal medullary (SAM) axis [31]. The vagus nerve plays an important role in initiating and perpetuating the relaxation response. Increase in vagal nerve activity (the tenth cranial nerve, which contains 75% of all parasympathetic fibers) works in several ways to decrease inflammation and enhance the immune function of many organ systems, including the skin [32]. The vagus nerve does this through the cholinergic anti-inflammatory pathway, which inhibits the release of cytokines. Some of the anti-inflammatory effects of MBTs include a decrease in C-reactive protein (CRP), interleukin-6, and tumor necrosis factor-alpha [26, 27].

Other reported effects of MBTs include beneficial effects on gene expression pathways in circulating immune cells [27], increased telomerase activity [33], and changes in the morphology of the brain responsible for emotional regulation [34].

In addition, MBTs have long-term benefits on some of the comorbidities of skin disorders, including depression, anxiety, shame, and social isolation [35]. Because MBTs have a broad effect on the psychological and spiritual aspects of disease, they also can help patients who are cured, but not healed. Many patients' "cured" acne can still leave noticeable scars, and patients with well-managed rosacea often have persistent erythema and telangiectasia.

MBTs also have been shown to reduce compulsive manipulation of skin lesions, especially in acne excoriée [36]. They also have been effective in other psychocutaneous disorders, including neurotic excoriations, trichotillomania, psychogenic pruritus, and neurodermatitis [35].

Interest and acceptance of MBTs in the general population is increasing. A survey of 2055 adults showed that 18.9%

of adults used at least one mind–body therapy in the previous year. On average, 40–50% of the respondents found that MBTs were "very helpful for their condition." Most of these therapies were done as self-care, with only 20.5% of them involving a visit to a provider [37].

Meditation Practices

Mindfulness Meditation

Meditation is the practice of intentionally bringing one's complete focus into the present moment, without judgment or emotional attachment, as a means to rest the mind and reach a state of consciousness that is different from our normal waking state. Meditation is not about clearing the mind, but rather gaining insight into the mind's patterns by being open and curious with attention to what is present. Cultivating this state of mind has been shown to reduce stress, anxiety [38], and depression [39], moderate pain [40], improve cognitive function [41], and even create changes in gray matter density [42] in regions of the brain related to emotional regulation, self-awareness, learning, and memory.

Mindfulness meditation has shown benefits for stress reduction in the field of dermatology when introduced in the 1990s by Jon Kabat-Zinn. Although performed with psoriasis patients, Kabat-Zinn's research supports that stress reduction techniques, including visualization of the therapeutic process and meditation, may be helpful in the treatment of skin disorders and can positively influence physiological factors in disease for patients actively engaged in implementing them.

Relaxation Response

Introduced by Dr. Herbert Benson in the 1960s, this form of meditation is described as a physical state of deep relaxation that engages the parasympathetic nervous system. When practiced regularly, it contributes to lower stress levels, increases well-being, and counteracts the physiological effects of stress and the fight-or-flight response, including reduction in blood pressure and resting heart rate [43]. It is performed by sitting in a quiet place, with eyes closed, and letting your muscles loosen and relax, starting with your feet and working upward with progressive muscular relaxation while breathing evenly through your nose, becoming aware of the breath, and repeating the word “one” with each exhalation. Research has shown that regular use of the relaxation response can help any health problem that is caused or exacerbated by chronic stress, which would include acne and rosacea [44].

Guided Imagery

Guided imagery involves the use of visualization techniques to elicit the somatosensory system to help the body enter a relaxed state. This technique can help with stress and anxiety by allowing the patient to manage negative emotions and visualize positive outcomes for their skin condition. Guided imagery can be used as a stand-alone practice, though it is often used in collaboration with other MBTs, including meditation, cognitive behavioral therapy (CBT), and hypnosis [4].

Autogenic Training

Autogenic training describes a technique similar to meditation, in which a series of statements is repeated about different parts of the body. The repetition of these statements is believed to influence the functioning of the autonomic nervous system, to aid in relaxation, and to help reduce symptoms of anxiety when combined with other forms of treatment. Although less well-known than other relaxation techniques such as progressive muscle relaxation and guided imagery, a meta-analytic study in 2008 found efficacy of autogenic training in the treatment of stress and anxiety [45].

Although specific studies correlating the use of meditation in acne and rosacea are lacking, evidence supports that meditation blunts the body's stress response by affecting the HPA axis and, ultimately, decreasing cortisol levels, or at least minimizing their increase in response to stress. A recent study regarding integrative mind–body training (IMBT) has shown that it can reduce salivary cortisol levels when compared to an equal amount of general relaxation time. This study also suggests that meditation or IMBT has a dose–response relationship, with a longer time spent meditating correlating with greater effect on cortisol levels. Addressing long-term stress and the associated elevation in cortisol can be beneficial in altering the onset and course of cutaneous conditions such as acne and rosacea [46].

Psychological Approaches

Biofeedback

Biofeedback is a technique that teaches patients to control involuntary bodily functions such as skin temperature, muscle tension, blood pressure, and heart rate to help manage stress. During biofeedback, patients are connected to electrical sensors which measure and provide auditory and visual feedback of these bodily processes to help them make subtle changes in their bodies to achieve the results they want [47]. By enhancing the patient's awareness of tension and helping them to relax, studies have shown biofeedback improves skin disorders that flare with stress or that have an autonomic nervous system component, including acne, eczema, psoriasis, and hyperhidrosis [4]. Through training, patients can learn how to consciously change the autonomic response and, with practice, may create new habit patterns [5, 44, 47].

Cognitive Behavioral Therapy

Cognitive behavioral therapy (CBT), as pioneered by Dr. Aaron Beck, is a short-term, goal-oriented psychotherapy treatment that helps patients understand and address dysfunctional thought patterns (cognitive) or actions (behavioral) that lead to skin damage or psychological distress. Methods used in CBT include habit reversal and aversion therapy and have been particularly useful in acne excoriée [35]. Each of these methods places a strong emphasis on "looking at the evidence" and replacing the patient's inaccurate automatic negative thoughts and behaviors that can contribute to and exacerbate emotional difficulties, depression, and anxiety with more accurate and desirable ones [48]. By becoming aware of the negative and often unrealistic thoughts that dampen their emotions and moods, patients are able to begin engaging in healthier thinking patterns, with a reduction in stress and anxiety. CBT has been combined with hypnosis, mindfulness, and other relaxation modalities to achieve positive outcomes [35].

Emotional Freedom Technique

Emotional freedom technique (EFT) combines elements of cognitive behavioral therapy(CBT), exposure therapy, and somatic stimulation using acupressure points. EFT is often called "tapping" because of this acupressure component. This technique focuses on selecting a specific negatively emotionally charged thought, memory, or problem area and repeating an affirmation such as "Even though I have this problem with symptom or diagnosis, I deeply and completely accept myself." This affirmation is continuously repeated by the patient while progressively tapping the finger on a series of up to 14 specific acupuncture sites on the head, chest, and hand [35].

EFT is thought to downregulate the activity of the limbic system, similar to acupuncture. Cortisol mediates limbic arousal. A study that measured salivary cortisol after EFT found that EFT reduced cortisol levels by 24%, which correlated with a statistically significant ($p < 0.05$) 58% decrease in anxiety scores [49]. Because anxiety and stress are so closely associated with acne and rosacea, EFT may be a useful adjunct to therapeutic regimens.

Hypnosis

Hypnosis, also referred to as hypnotherapy, uses guided relaxation, intense concentration, focused attention, and heightened suggestibility to help patients access information in their subconscious to change their behavior and thoughts. It has been proposed that hypnosis may make suggestions more effective by inhibiting competing thoughts so that the focus can be solely on the suggestion [35].

Both acne and rosacea have been found to benefit from hypnosis. The goal of hypnosis is to induce relaxation to help normalize the immune system through restoring autonomic, hormonal, and immune balance and giving the patient a sense of control. Hypnotic suggestions made to the patient are intended to help increase self-confidence, self-esteem, and problem-solving skills and optimize treatment outcomes [44].

Hypnosis can be performed alone or combined with various modalities, particularly CBT methods, to target the inflammatory aspects of acne; the subjective experience of anxiety, depression, shame, or embarrassment associated with having acne; as well as behaviors motivated by the acne such as squeezing, picking, and social withdrawal.

Because acne and rosacea can be triggered or aggravated by stress, incorporating MBT in the clinical setting as well as teaching patients how to implement them for self-care not only deserves more attention in treatment planning but may amplify treatment outcomes.

Breathwork

Breathwork is the purposeful control of the depth and rhythm of respiration. It can quickly produce beneficial mind–body states. In the United States, 10.9% of adults use deep breathing as a practice, primarily for stress relief [50].

Most breathwork practices are derived from pranayama, which is a branch of yoga. Pranayama can be translated as *Prana* (vital energy force) and *Yama* (control/regulation). In pranayama yoga, the practitioner controls the depth, force, and duration of (1) inhalation (2) and exhalation, (3) the amount of time the breath is held, and (4) the time between breaths. There are many variations of these four steps, each attempting to create a particular desirable mind–body state [51].

The most effective pranayama breathing technique for stress reduction is decreasing the rate of respiration, utilizing deep diaphragmatic breaths, and increasing the duration of expiration [52]. This technique rapidly activates the parasympathetic nervous system via stimulation of the vagus nerve, the tenth cranial nerve which connects the brain and visceral organs with afferent and efferent nerves.

This shift to enhanced parasympathetic activity results in overall stress reduction and reduction in inflammation [53]. In a meta-analysis of clinical patients, pranayama along with asana (pose) practice was shown to reduce C-reactive protein and IL-6 and has an antioxidant effect in response to oxidative stress [54]. In addition, increased leukocyte telomere length was noted [55]. Telomeres are located at the tips of chromosomes and protect cellular DNA. Unstable telomeres have been linked to a wide range of age- and stress-induced physical and mental disorders.

Chanting, singing, vocal toning [56], and humming, all of which involve a rapid inhalation and prolonged exhalation accompanied by vibration of the vocal cords, are other practices which stimulate the parasympathetic nervous system. Chanting "OM" or "One" can quickly induce the relaxation response via the upregulation of the parasympathetic nervous system [43]. Vocal toning, which typically involves using an open vowel sound with a prolonged expiration, has a similar effect.

Movement

Qi Gong and Tai Chi

To understand the ancient Chinese practices Qi Gong and Tai Chi, one must first understand the concept of Qi (pronounced "chi") [57]. It has been compared with the electrical charge in a battery; when the battery is old, the body tires easily, and when the battery is charged, one can be active without fatigue [58]. If a person can tap into their inner Qi, they can channel this energy to stimulate a multitude of physiological components that can benefit their overall health [57, 59]. These components include, but are not limited to, lymphatic, immunologic, cardiovascular, neuronal, endocrinologic, psychologic, and musculoskeletal systems [59, 60]. Qi Gong and Tai Chi are special meditative forms of exercise that utilize movement, meditation, and breathwork to reduce stress and promote relaxation through their physiological influence on the body's systems through the use of Qi [58, 61–63].

Randomized controlled trials and systematic reviews have shown that both of these practices have a comparably positive relationship in stress reduction and relaxation. This stress reduction is predominantly driven by activation of the parasympathetic nervous system and the attenuation of the sympathetic nervous system [59, 60, 64]. Tai Chi and Qi Gong have been documented to reduce anxiety as well as improve mood disorders such as depression and anxiety [60, 61, 64]. Aside from stress reduction and mood enhancement benefits, these practices have also been shown to reduce pro-inflammatory markers such as interleukin-6, which have been documented to play a pathophysiologic role in acne [65].

Yoga

Yoga is an ancient practice that originated in India thousands of years ago; it combines physical postures, controlled breathing, and meditation [66]. Despite its long history, only in recent years has yoga become one of the most popular alternative MBTs [67].

Many studies have demonstrated the positive effect of the practice of yoga on health, including both physiological and psychological benefits [66]. Yoga has been shown to reduce stress and anxiety via an increased vagal tone, increased gamma-aminobutyric acid (GABA) levels, and promotion of frontal alpha wave activity, which improves relaxation [66]. In addition to influencing the stress response, yoga has been shown to influence neurotransmitters, oxidative stress, lipids, and growth factors in a manner similar to antidepressants and psychotherapy [68]. Yoga has also shown the added benefit of reducing systemic inflammation in the body by decreasing circulating levels of interleukin-6, C-reactive protein, and cortisol [69], factors that play a role in moderate to severe acne [70].

Those who practice yoga with consistency have shown improved responses to acute stressors in comparison to those who do not have a regular practice. Furthermore, participants of yoga had more self-efficacy and confidence in being able to overcome daily stressors. Similarly, those who practice yoga showed an improved quality of sleep, feeling more rested the next day. Yoga has shown many benefits to those who suffer with skin conditions such as acne and rosacea, including improved ability to respond to stress, decreased inflammation, better sleep, and higher quality of life, making it a worthwhile adjunct to conventional therapy.

Body Work

Acupuncture and Acupressure

Acupuncture is part of traditional Chinese medicine (TCM; see Chap. 11 for more details). One of the principles of TCM is the restoration of the balance of energy (chi) flow within the body. Chi flows along longitudinally oriented meridians on the surface of the body. In acupuncture, stainless steel needles are inserted into specific points along these meridians. The needles are 0.10–0.25 mm in diameter and are inserted 1/4–1/2 inch beneath the skin surface.

Acupuncture has been used for a wide range of inflammatory and infectious skin diseases [71]. Two systematic reviews of the use of acupuncture do reveal some promising results in acne. A 2018 review included ten randomized trials of various acupuncture techniques on acne [72]. The results showed that the chance of achieving a >30% and >50 improvement in lesion count was the same in the acupuncture-treated group and the standard pharmacotherapy groups. The acupuncture groups reported fewer adverse events. Another 2013 review evaluated 43 trials with 3453 patients, and it did show improvement in acne in various forms of acupuncture combined with herbal medications [73]. However, both reviews cited poor study quality as an issue.

A case report of acupuncture for rosacea showed clearing of rosacea after three sessions of acupuncture [74]. Doppler studies suggested that this was due to improved vascular microcirculation.

The biomedical mechanism of action for the effect of acupuncture on acne is unknown. But it may have an effect on the reduction of inflammation via the innate and adaptive immune networks and the muscarinic acetylcholine receptors [72]. Acupuncture also increases the level of peripheral beta-endorphins, enkephalins, serotonin, norepinephrine, gamma-aminobutyric acid (GABA), and oxytocin, which are related to its effects on pain and mood [75, 76].

In a 2018 Cochrane review, acupuncture was found to have a beneficial effect in depression [77], and a 2019 systematic review found a benefit in anxiety [78]. Therefore, acupuncture may also have a place in dealing with depression and anxiety, which can be issues in patients with acne and rosacea.

Reiki

Reiki is a relatively modern technique, created by a Japanese monk in the 1920s. The recharging and balancing of subtle universal life energy (ki) in the body is an underlying principle of Reiki. Reiki is done by lightly laying hands on or just above the surface of the skin. In some forms of Reiki, the hands are lightly placed on chakras, which are centers of energy. In other forms, the hands are placed in symptomatic areas. The recipient of Reiki is fully clothed and may be prone or seated.

Three recent reviews of Reiki have shown promising results in the domains of mental and physical symptoms. These include induction of the relaxation response [79]; reduction of pain, anxiety, and depression; and improved quality of life in patients with various physical disorders [80, 81].

Massage Therapy

Massage therapy has a long history of use in hospitalized patients and in nonmedical settings. It is often used for relief of pain in musculoskeletal disorders and for relief of stress and anxiety. It may also benefit patients who may feel stigmatized, ashamed, and isolated because of the appearance of their skin. There are many varieties of massage, but Swedish massage is among the most popular and researched technique. In Swedish massage, the skin and underlying structures such as muscles, tendons, and fascia are firmly kneaded in long strokes.

Studies have demonstrated many beneficial effects of massage, including increased levels of oxytocin, dopamine, and natural killer cells and decreased levels of adrenocorticotropic hormone (ACTH) and nitric oxide [82]. Another study looked at the effect of single-session Swedish massage on the immune system of healthy adults [83]. It found increased number of circulating CD-4, CD-8, CD-25, and CD-56 + lymphocytes and decreased levels of cytokines IL-4, IL-10, and IL-13, which can contribute to inflammation in the body, including the skin.

Community and Connection

It may seem like the patient in our examination room is an autonomous individual, not affected by connections to the outside world. But in reality, all of us live in a web of connections. These connections can support us in coping with the many stressors of daily life, including illness.

Support Groups

The psychological issues that are the result of having visible facial lesions are well documented, and they often result in peoples' avoidance of social interactions. There is an emerging online body-positive movement that supports people with all forms of visible body issues [84]. Most patients with acne are in the age group that heavily utilizes social media, and these online support groups are a place where many personal connections are made. It is important to refer patients with significant mental health issues to an appropriate provider.

Spirituality

The mental and physical health benefits of connections to one's spiritual life and spiritual community have been studied extensively. A study of 149 patients with skin disease (scleroderma, systemic lupus erythematosus, and melanoma) showed that spirituality decreased levels of depression and anxiety [85]. The dimensions of spirituality that seemed to be the most impactful were hope for a better future and feeling connected to the universe. Reviews of the literature have confirmed the beneficial effects of religion and spirituality in a wide range of physical and mental disorders including cancer, HIV/AIDS, burns, and chronic pain [86]. Some of the explanations for this effect include improved coping skills, enhanced social interactions, and assistance within a religious community.

Creative Therapy

Creative therapy serves as an umbrella term for a variety of techniques that are both artistic and expressive in nature. These techniques include, but are not limited to, journaling, music, and art.

The use of music in medicine can be classified as either *music medicine* or *music therapy*, the former being administered by a healthcare professional and the latter by a music therapist. Music medicine encompasses medical personnel providing pre-recorded music to the patient for passive listening [87]. Music therapy includes active listening (live music), improvising, composing, participating (instrumentally or vocally), and/or a combination of these modalities [87]. Music therapy is regarded as a more effective strategy because a music therapist can more actively engage with the patient through an individualized intervention [87]. Regardless of the approach, both methods have been shown to influence the patient's psychological, physical, social, and spiritual health. Patients reported reduced anxiety and exhibited a lower resting heart rate, respiratory rate, and systolic blood pressure [87]. Patients also exhibited improvement in their communication skills, both verbal and nonverbal, and an improvement in their overall quality of life [87].

Writing interventions, which are simple and inexpensive practices, benefit patients like those dealing with acne and rosacea who may suffer from body image-related concerns, especially if one uses a self-compassion-focused prompt [88]. Self-compassion is the capacity to adopt a kind, caring attitude toward oneself in times of difficulty. It is a mindset shift that has been linked to reduced psychological distress. Emerging evidence shows that this model of treatment enhances one's cognitive flexibility, adaptability to life changes, and coping mechanisms, which can lead to lower rates of stress and depression over one's body image [88]. This method is particularly beneficial for those with high self-judgment and low self-compassion [88].

Art therapy is a cost-effective psychological therapy that may be more beneficial for adult and pediatric populations who struggle with talk therapy. Art therapy can include, but is not limited to, painting, clay work, and creative digital media. Art can help an individual achieve a greater understanding of themselves as well as enhance their expression of feelings. Studies on art have also shown potential benefits such as decreased anxiety, depression, trauma, and distress while increasing cognitive function, improving coping mechanisms, and increasing quality of life [89].

References

1. Chen Y, Lyga J. Brain-skin connection: stress, inflammation and skin aging. Inflamm Allergy Drug Targets. 2014;13(3):177–90.
2. Honeyman JF. Psychoneuroimmunology and the skin. Acta Derm Venereol. 2016;217:38–46.
3. Rainer BM, Kang S, Chien AL. Rosacea: epidemiology, pathogenesis, and treatment. Dermato-endocrinology. 2017;9(1):e1361574.
4. Hughes H, Brown BW, Lawlis GF, Fulton JE Jr. Treatment of acne vulgaris by biofeedback relaxation and cognitive imagery. J Psychosom Res. 1983;27:185–91.
5. Shenefelt P. Psychological interventions in the management of common skin conditions. Psychol Res Behav Manag. 2010;3:51–63.
6. Gieler U, Gieler T, Kupfer JP. Acne and quality of life - impact and management. J Eur Acad Dermatol Venereol. 2015;29(Suppl 4):12–4.
7. Balkrishnan R, McMichael AJ, Hu JY, Camacho FT, Shew KR, Bouloc A, et al. Correlates of health-related quality of life in women with severe facial blemishes. Int J Dermatol. 2006;45:111–5.
8. Ritvo E, Rosso JQ, Stillman MA, Riche C. Psychosocial judgements and perceptions of adolescents with acne vulgaris: a blinded, controlled comparison of adult and peer evaluations. Biopsychosoc Med. 2011;5:11.
9. Timms RM. Moderate acne as a potential barrier to social relationships: myth or reality? Psychol Health Med. 2013;18:310–20.
10. Halvorsen JA, Stern RS, Dalgard F, Thoresen M, Bjertness E, Lien L. Suicidal ideation, mental health problems, and social impairment are increased in adolescents with acne: a population-based study. J Invest Dermatol. 2011;131:363–70.
11. Jones-Caballero M, Chren MM, Soler B, Pedrosa E, Peñas PF. Quality of life in mild to moderate acne: relationship to clinical severity and factors influencing change with treatment. J Eur Acad Dermatol Venereol. 2007;21:219–26.

12. Demircay Z, Seckin D, Senol A, Demir F. Patient's perspective: an important issue not to be overlooked in assessing acne severity. Eur J Dermatol. 2008;18:181–4.
13. Dreno B, Alirezai M, Auffret N, Beylot C, Chivot M, Daniel F, et al. Clinical and psychological correlation in acne: use of the ECLA and CADI scales. Ann Dermatol Venereol. 2007;134:451–5.
14. Yazici K, Baz K, Yazici AE, Köktürk A, Tot S, Demirseren D, et al. Disease-specific quality of life is associated with anxiety and depression in patients with acne. J Eur Acad Dermatol Venereol. 2004;18:435–9.
15. Dalgard FJ, Gieler U, Tomas-Aragones L, Lien L, Poot F, Jemec GBE, et al. The psychological burden of skin diseases: a cross-sectional multicenter study among dermatological out-patients in 13 European Countries. J Invest Dermatol. 2015;135(4):984–91.
16. Cunliffe WJ. Acne and unemployment. Br J Dermatol. 1986;115:386.
17. Krejci-Manwaring J, Kerchner K, Feldman SR, Rapp DA, Rapp SR. Social sensitivity and acne: the role of personality in negative social consequences and quality of life. Int J Psychiatry Med. 2006;36:121–30.
18. Oussedik E, Bourcier M, Tan J. Psychosocial burden and other impacts of rosacea on patients' quality of life. Dermatol Clin. 2018;36(2):103–13.
19. Chiu A, Chon SY, Kimball AB. The response of skin disease to stress: changes in the severity of acne vulgaris as affected by examination stress. Arch Dermatol. 2003;139(7):897–900.
20. Orion E, Wolf R. Psychologic factors in the development of facial dermatoses. Clin Dermatol. 2014;32(6):763–6.
21. Elenkov IJ, Webster EL, Torpy DJ, Chrousos GP. Stress, corticotropin-releasing hormone, glucocorticoids, and the immune/inflammatory response: acute and chronic effects. Ann N Y Acad Sci. 1999;876:1–11.
22. Slominski A, Wortsman J, Tuckey RC, Paus R. Differential expression of HPA axis homolog in the skin. Mol Cell Endocrinol. 2007;265–266:143–9.
23. Toyoda M, Morohashi M. Pathogenesis of acne. Med Electron Microsc. 2001;34:29–40.
24. Alexopoulos A, Chrousos GP. Stress-related skin disorders. Rev Endocr Metab Disord. 2016;17:295.

25. Zari S, Alrahmani D. The association between stress and acne among female medical students in Jeddah, Saudi Arabia. Clin Cosmet Investig Dermatol. 2017;10:503–6.
26. Morgan N, Irwin MR, Chung M, Wang C. The effects of mind-body therapies on the immune system: meta-analysis. PLoS One. 2014;9(7):e100903.
27. Bower JE, Irwin MR. Mind-body therapies and control of inflammatory biology: a descriptive review. Brain Behav Immun. 2016;51:1–11.
28. Muehsam D, Lutgendorf S, Mills PJ, Rickhi B, Chevalier G, Bat N, et al. The embodied mind: a review on functional genomic and neurological correlates of mind-body therapies. Neurosci Biobehav Rev. 2017;73:165–81.
29. Stahl JE, Dossett ML, LaJoie AS, Denninger JW, Mehta DH, Goldman R, et al. Relaxation response and resiliency training and its effect on healthcare resource utilization. PLoS One. 2015;10(10):e0140212.
30. Dhabhar FS. Psychological stress and immunoprotection versus immunopathology in the skin. Clin Dermatol. 2013;31(1):18–30.
31. Dusek JA, Benson H. Mind-body medicine: a model of the comparative clinical impact of the acute stress and relaxation responses. Minn Med. 2009;92(5):47–50.
32. Breit S, Kupferberg A, Rogler G, Hasler G. Vagus nerve as modulator of the brain–gut axis in psychiatric and inflammatory disorders. Front Psych. 2018;9:44–59.
33. Schutte NS, Malouff JM. A meta-analytic review of the effects of mindfulness meditation on telomerase activity. Psychoneuroendocrinology. 2014;42:45–8.
34. Marchand WR. Mindfulness-based stress reduction, mindfulness-based cognitive therapy, and Zen meditation for depression, anxiety, pain, and psychological distress. J Psychiatr Pract. 2012;18(4):233–52.
35. Shenefelt PD. Psychodermatological disorders: recognition and treatment. Int J Dermatol. 2011;50(11):1309–22.
36. Shenefelt PD. Using hypnosis to facilitate resolution of psychogenic excoriations in acne excoriée. Am J Clin Hypn. 2004;46(3):239–45.
37. Wolsko PM, Eisenberg DM, Davis RB, Phillips RS. Use of mind-body medical therapies. J Gen Intern Med. 2004;19(1):43–50.
38. Kim B, Lee SH, Kim YW, Choi TK, Yook K, Suh SY, et al. Effectiveness of a mindfulness-based cognitive therapy program

as an adjunct to pharmacotherapy in patients with panic disorder. J Anxiety Disord. 2010;24(6):590–5.
39. Godfrin KA, van Heeringen C. The effects of mindfulness-based cognitive therapy on recurrence of depressive episodes, mental health and quality of life: a randomized controlled study. Behav Res Ther. 2010;48(8):738–46.
40. Zeidan F, Martucci KT, Kraft RA, Gordon NS, McHaffie JG, Coghill RC. Brain mechanisms supporting the modulation of pain by mindfulness meditation. J Neurosci. 2011;14:5540–8.
41. Zeidan F, Johnson SK, Diamond BJ, David Z, Goolkasian P. Mindfulness meditation improves cognition: evidence of brief mental training. Conscious Cogn. 2010;2:597–605.
42. Hölzel BK, Carmody J, Vangel M, Congleton C, Yerramsetti SM, Gard T, et al. Mindfulness practice leads to increases in regional brain gray matter density. Psychiatry Res. 2011;191(1):36–43.
43. Benson H, Klipper MZ. The relaxation response. New York: Avon; 1975.
44. Schenefelt P. Biofeedback, cognitive-behavioral methods, and hypnosis in dermatology: it is all in your mind? Dermatol Ther. 2003;16:114–22.
45. Manzoni GM, Pagnini F, Castelnuovo G, Molinari E. Relaxation training for anxiety: a ten-years systematic review with meta-analysis. BMC Psychiatry. 2008;8:41.
46. Veerkamp P, Mousdicas N, Bednarek R. Rosacea fulminans precipitated by acute stress: a case report describing an integrative approach for a patient reluctant to use isotretinoin. Integr Med (Encinitas). 2016;15(6):32–5.
47. Fried RG, Hussain SH. Nonpharmacological management of common skin and psychocutaneous disorders. Dermatol Ther. 2008;21:60–8.
48. Hofmann SG, Asnaani A, Vonk IJ, Sawyer AT, Fang A. The efficacy of cognitive behavioral therapy: a review of meta-analyses. Cognit Ther Res. 2012;36(5):427–44.
49. Clond M. Emotional freedom techniques for anxiety: a systematic review with meta-analysis. J Nerv Ment Dis. 2016;204(5):388–95.
50. Clarke TC, Back LI, Stussman BJ, Barnes PM, Nahin RL. Trends in the use of complementary health approaches among adults: United States. 2002–2012. National health statistics reports: no 79. Hyattsville: National Center for Health Statistics; 2015.
51. Saoji AA, Raghavendra BR, Manjunath NK. Effects of yogic breath regulation: a narrative review of scientific evidence. J Ayurveda Integr Med. 2019;10(1):50–8.

52. Jerath R, Edry JW, Barnes VA, Jerath V. Physiology of long pranayamic breathing: neural respiratory elements may provide a mechanism that explains how slow deep breathing shifts the autonomic nervous system. Med Hypotheses. 2006;67(3):566–71.
53. Kuppusamy M, Kamaldeen D, Pitani R, Amaldas J, Shanmugam P. Effects of Bhramari Pranayama on health -a systematic review. J Tradit Complement Med. 2018;8(1):11–6.
54. Mohammad A, Thakur P, Kumar R, Kaur S, Saini RV, Saini AK. Biological markers for the effects of yoga as a complementary and alternative medicine. J Complement Integr Med. 2019;16(1):1–15.
55. Rathore M, Abraham J. Implication of asana, pranayama and meditation on telomere stability. Int J Yoga. 2018;11(3):186–93.
56. Snow S, Bernardi NF, Sabet-Kassouf N, Moran D, Lehmann A. Exploring the experience and effects of vocal toning. J Music Ther. 2018;55(2):221–50.
57. Jahnke R, Larkey L, Rogers C, Etnier J, Lin F. A comprehensive review of health benefits of qigong and tai chi. Am J Health Promot. 2010;24(6):e1–e25.
58. Chu DA. Tai chi, qi gong and reiki. Phys Med Rehabil Clin N Am. 2004;15(4):773–81.
59. Lee M, Soo Lee M, Kim H, Moon S. Qigong reduced blood pressure and catecholamine levels of patients with essential hypertension. Int J Neurosci. 2003;113:1691.
60. Tai H-C, Chou Y-S, Tzeng I-S, Wei C-Y, Su C-H, Liu W-C, et al. Effect of tai chi synergy T1 exercise on autonomic function, metabolism, and physical fitness of healthy individuals. Evid Based Complement Alternat Med. 2018;2018:6351938.
61. Matos LC, Sousa CM, Gonçalves M, Gabriel J, Machado J, Greten HJ. Qigong as a traditional vegetative biofeedback therapy: long-term conditioning of physiological mind-body effects. Biomed Res Int. 2015;2015:531789.
62. Jalalat S. Yoga for dermatologic conditions. Cutis. 2015;95(4):E23–5.
63. Wang F, E-KO L, Wu T, Benson H, Fricchione G, Wang W, et al. The effects of tai chi on depression, anxiety, and psychological well-being: a systematic review and meta-analysis. Int J Behav Med. 2014;21(4):605–17.
64. Tsai J-C, Wang W-H, Chan P, Lin LJ, Wang CH, Tomlinson B, et al. The beneficial effects of Tai Chi Chuan on blood pressure and lipid profile and anxiety in a randomized controlled trial. J Altern Complement Med. 2003;9:747–54.

65. Chen HH, Yeh ML, Lee FY. The effects of baduanjin qigong in the prevention of bone loss for middle-aged women. Am J Chin Med. 2006;34:741–7.
66. Jeter PE, Slutsky J, Singh N, Khalsa SBS. Yoga as a therapeutic intervention: a bibliometric analysis of published research studies from 1967 to 2013. J Altern Complement Med. 2015;21(10):586–92.
67. National Center for Complementary and Integrative Health. The use of complementary and alternative medicine in the United States. U.S. Department of Health and Human Services; 2017.
68. Balasubramaniam M, Telles S, Doraiswamy PM. Yoga on our minds: a systematic review of yoga for neuropsychiatric disorders. Front Psych. 2012;3:117.
69. Kiecolt-Glaser JK, Christian L, Preston H, Houts CR, Malarkey WB, Emery CF, et al. Stress, inflammation, and yoga practice. Psychosom Med. 2010;72(2):113–21.
70. Namazi MR, Parhizkar AR, Jowkar F. Serum levels of hypersensitive-C-reactive protein in moderate and severe acne. Indian Dermatol Online J. 2015;6(4):253–7.
71. Iliev E. Acupuncture in dermatology. Clin Dermatol. 1998;16(6):659–88.
72. Mansu SSY, Liang H, Parker S, Coyle ME, Wang K, Zhang AL, et al. Acupuncture for acne vulgaris: a systematic review and meta-analysis. Evid Based Complement Alternat Med. 2018;2018:4806734.
73. Cao H-J, Yang G-Y, Wang Y-Y, Liu J-P. Acupoint stimulation for acne: a systematic review of randomized controlled trials. Med Acupunct. 2013;25(3):173–94.
74. Gao Y, Lin W, Zhou S, Shi G, He J, Chen Y. Treatment of rosacea using acupuncture for improving the local skin microcirculation: a case report. Medicine. 2018;97(34):e11931.
75. Gabriella H. Biomedical effects of acupuncture. Int J Complement Altern Med. 2015;2(1):1–5.
76. Malizia E, Andreucci G, Paolucci D, Crescenzi F, Fabbri A, Fraioli F. Electroacupuncture and peripheral beta-endorphin and ACTH levels. Lancet. 1979;2(8141):535–6.
77. Smith CA, Armour M, Lee MS, Wang L-Q, Hay PJ. Acupuncture for depression. Cochrane Database Syst Rev. 2018;3(3):CD004046.

78. Li M, Xing X, Yao L, Li X, He W, Wang M, et al. Acupuncture for treatment of anxiety, an overview of systematic reviews. Complement Ther Med. 2019;43:247–52.
79. McManus DE. Reiki is better than placebo and has broad potential as a complementary health therapy. J Evid Based Complement Alternat Med. 2017;22(4):1051–7.
80. Doğan M. The effect of reiki on pain: a meta-analysis. Complement Ther Clin Pract. 2018;31:384–7.
81. Billot M, Daycard M, Wood C, Tchalla A. Reiki therapy for pain, anxiety and quality of life. BMJ Support Palliat Care. 2019;9:434–8.
82. Morhenn V, Beavin LE, Zak PJ. Massage increases oxytocin and reduces adrenocorticotropin hormone in humans. Altern Ther Health Med. 2012;18(6):11–8.
83. Rapaport MH, Schettler P, Bresee C. A preliminary study of the effects of a single session of Swedish massage on hypothalamic–pituitary–adrenal and immune function in normal individuals. J Altern Complement Med. 2010;16(10):1079–88.
84. Cohen R, Irwin L, Newton-John T, Slater A. #bodypositivity: a content analysis of body positive accounts on Instagram. Body Image. 2019;29:47–57.
85. Unterrainer H-F, Lukanz M, Pilch M, Scharf S, Glawischnig-Goschnik M, Wutte N, et al. Spirituality and mood pathology in severe skin conditions: a prospective observational study. Arch Dermatol Res. 2016;308(7):521–5.
86. Siegel K, Anderman SJ, Schrimshaw EW. Religion and coping with health-related stress. Psychol Health. 2001;16(6):631–53.
87. Bradt J, Dileo C, Potvin N. Music for stress and anxiety reduction in coronary heart disease patients. Cochrane Database Syst Rev. 2013;12:CD006577.
88. Przezdziecki A, Alcorso J, Sherman KA. My changed body: background, development and acceptability of a self-compassion based writing activity for female survivors of breast cancer. Patient Educ Couns. 2016;99(5):870–4.
89. Uttley L, Stevenson M, Scope A, Rawdin A, Sutton A. The clinical and cost effectiveness of group art therapy for people with non-psychotic mental health disorders: a systematic review and cost-effectiveness analysis. BMC Psychiatry. 2015;15:151.

Chapter 9
Functional Medicine Approaches

Michelle Jeffries, Matthew Goldberg and Valori Treloar

The doctor of the future will give no medication, but will interest his patients in the care of the human frame, diet and in the cause and prevention of disease.

—*Thomas A. Edison*

Introduction: What Is Functional Medicine?

Functional medicine is a comprehensive science-based approach to optimize health and wellness. It focuses on the therapeutic partnership between the patient and clinician to unveil patterns and connections to the deeper root causes of health concerns.

The patterns of underlying health issues can be evaluated in a systems-based approach focused on seven systems of clinical imbalances: assimilation/gastrointestinal, immune, energy, detoxification, cardiovascular/lymphatic, hormones/neurotransmitter, and musculoskeletal/cellular structure:

M. Jeffries (✉)
Private Practice, Scottsdale, AZ, USA

M. Goldberg
Department of Dermatology, Icahn School of Medicine at Mount Sinai, New York, NY, USA

V. Treloar
Integrative Dermatology, Newton, MA, USA

R. N. Rupani, P. A. Lio (eds.), *Integrative Dermatology*,
https://doi.org/10.1007/978-3-030-58954-7_9

- *Assimilation/gastrointestinal system*: The gastrointestinal system is focused on how our body consumes, assimilates, absorbs, and utilizes nutrients throughout the digestive system. The gut microbiome and intestinal permeability also play roles.
- *Immune system*: The immune system is involved in defending against potentially harmful entities and assists in repairing damage to cells, tissues, and organs. It is also involved in the repair process of healing. Dysfunction can result in disturbances in immune tolerance.
- *Energy system*: The energy system is how the body utilizes fuel sources for energy and how the body conserves or expends energy. It focuses on mitochondrial health and function.
- *Detoxification system*: The detoxification systems transform potential toxins into inert by-products and how our body eliminates them.
- *Cardiovascular and lymphatic transport systems*: The cardiovascular and lymphatic systems focus on how the body moves and transports nutrients throughout the body, as well as the movement of white blood cells throughout the body.
- *Hormone and neurotransmitter systems*: The hormone and neurotransmitter systems are involved in how the body communicates and sends messages and signals.
- *Musculoskeletal system and cellular structure*: The musculoskeletal system and cellular structures are how the body functions as a structure. Bone density, muscle strength, fascial connections, cutaneous barrier function, and the integrity of the membrane structures of the body are included in this section.

To explore how these seven clinical imbalances play a personalized role in health and wellness in more detail, functional medicine uses various tools such as an in-depth physical examination, symptom questionnaires, laboratory tests, genetics, etc. The information gathered is reviewed with the patient in detail, and together the clinician and patient set goals and priorities of how to optimize the patient's health. The next step is the implementation of a therapeutic treatment plan.

Therapeutic treatments from a functional medicine approach focus on addressing the core imbalances by blending prescription treatments and lifestyle changes. The main two questions that are addressed when deciding on a therapeutic focus are: Does this patient need to get rid of something? Does this patient have an unmet need for optimal function? The answers to these questions help determine the focus of personalized lifestyle changes. The areas of lifestyle changes are:

- Sleep and relaxation
- Exercise and movement
- Nutrition (food, vitamins, minerals, supplements, botanicals, etc.)
- Stress management
- Relationships and community connections
- Environmental factors (quality of air, water, etc.)
- Mental factors (cognition, perception, and psychosocial factors)
- Emotional factors (awareness and regulation of emotions)
- Spiritual connections (sense of purpose and meaning)

With collaboration between the patient and clinician, the functional medicine approach results in a personalized comprehensive therapeutic approach to healing and optimizing health. Next we will dive deeper into how the functional medicine approach can be applied to acne and rosacea.

Functional Medicine Approach to Acne and Rosacea

The focus of this chapter is to illustrate the functional medicine approach to acne and rosacea. Clinicians know that diseases are multifactorial and that patients are different and vary in response to our protocols. We see it every day in practice. Functional medicine allows us to begin to dissect this by addressing acne and rosacea through the seven clinical imbalances in the functional medicine matrix. Each of the seven clinical imbalances will be briefly reviewed within the context of acne and/or rosacea, and a brief summary of therapeutic treatment options will be discussed.

Assimilation/Gastrointestinal System

Of all skin diseases, rosacea is the one that dermatology has always considered to be affected by diet. No single food impacts all rosacea patients, but the standard of care includes journaling to identify possible triggers: foods, beverages, weather conditions, emotions, and activity [1]. On the other hand, as recently as 2011, the American Academy of Dermatology proclaimed that diet had no impact on acne [2]. The dogma relied largely on two studies from 1969 [3] to 1971 [4] which we now know to have major flaws. Only recently have researchers delved into this realm again and, this time around, the results are very different.

Dairy [5] and a high-glycemic load diet [6] clearly trigger or exacerbate acne in most of those with a genetic susceptibility to the disease. Melnik has written extensively on the presumed mechanism for the dairy and GL effects [7].

Insulin appears to be a prime mover in acne. Both insulin and IGF-1 appear to impair FOX01 suppression of the androgen receptor, PPAR gamma, LXR alpha, and SREBP1, with resultant increase in sebum, hyperkeratosis, and inflammation [8]. Insulin resistance rises during puberty, which is not surprising, as it is one of the growth hormones [9]. The arc describing the adolescent rise and fall of insulin resistance traces the arc of acne appearance and resolution over the same period [10].

"Glycemic load" (GL) describes the level and rate of rise of blood sugar in response to a given food. Foods with a high GL result in high and fast rises in blood sugar. Those with a low GL do the opposite. Insulin tracks blood sugar, so foods with a high GL tend to have a high insulinemic load (IL) as well. Intake of high GL/IL foods results in higher overall insulin levels pushing inflammatory physiology.

The rate of food intake affects blood sugar/insulin response. Sugary drinks consumed slowly over a longer period of time trigger a lower insulin response than when ingested over a few minutes. To improve physiologic inflammation, eat slowly [11].

In 1983, *Archives of Dermatology* contained the following observation: "... several highly-motivated patients with acne ... had a rapid, indeed almost abrupt, clearing of their acne through correction of faulty bowel elimination by means of a daily serving of 30 g of an "all-bran" breakfast cereal" [12]. A publication in *Metabolism* in 1995 elucidates the mechanism for such acne improvement with a high-fiber breakfast: "High fiber meals were associated with a significant reduction in postprandial serum glucose and insulin" [13].

Dissociation of the glycemic and insulinemic responses to milk may help explain why dairy exacerbates or triggers acne in susceptible patients. The glycemic response to full-fat dairy is not pronounced, but surprisingly, the insulin response resembles that seen with sugar [14]. Given that cow's milk is designed to support growth of calves, and that insulin is one of the growth hormones, insulin elevation should not be unexpected with milk intake.

Milk also raises IGF-1 and makes it more biologically available by lowering its binding protein [15]. Those with the genetic disease Laron syndrome—characterized by very short stature, facial dysmorphism, obesity, and delayed puberty—have an inability to generate IGF-1. They only develop acne when given extrinsic IGF-1 supplementation [16].

In the future, we will look back on rosacea as our gateway to the discovery of the gastrointestinal microbiome's impact on skin disease. Small intestine bacterial overgrowth (SIBO) appears to be one of the triggers for rosacea. Treatment of SIBO reduces/eliminates rosacea. When SIBO recurs, rosacea returns [17]. Botanical antimicrobials combined with a low GL or a low fermentable oligosaccharides, disaccharides, monosaccharides, and polyols (FODMAP) diet may be more effective than antibiotics for SIBO [18]. Treatment of SIBO tends to also alter colonic flora whose role is less clear, but likely to be even more profound. Recent work on colonic flora and its impact on immune function suggest that this will become a central focus of therapeutic intervention for diseases that have elements of autoimmune dysfunction [19].

Even a 24-h dietary recall by the patient gives the functional medicine doctor a view into paths for intervention. With a thorough understanding of the mechanisms by which dairy and a high-GL diet impact the pathophysiology of acne (and the acneiform aspects of rosacea), the physician can better educate the patient about the reasons and options for altering diet and decreasing acne activity.

Immune System

Melnik elegantly diagrammed the "inflammasomopathy" of acne triggered by diet. His increasingly supported theory explains why overgrowth of *Cutibacterium* (previously known as *Propionobacterium*) *acnes*, a normal inhabitant of the follicle that protects against pathogens such as *Staphylococcus aureus*, becomes part of the pathogenic process of acne. Suppression of FOX01 and mTORC by insulin/IGF-1 permits increased sebum production and follicular hyperkeratosis—feeding the bacteria and optimizing anaerobic conditions for growth. The same mechanism ramps up androgen receptor activation and inflammation [20]. As discussed in the preceding section, dietary change to decrease GL/IL decreases inflammation.

Inflammation is an oxidative process; intracellular reactive oxygen species rise with activation of transcription factors like Nfkb, AP1, and kinases like JAK/STAT [21]. Oxidative stress is high in acne [22]. In severe acne, activity of the antioxidant enzyme, superoxide dismutase, is decreased [23]. Levels of the antioxidants zinc and vitamin A are both low in those with acne compared to those without [24, 25].

With the advent of isotretinoin, supplementation with vitamin A has not been explored. In spite of documentation that low levels of zinc correspond to increased acne, supplementation with zinc has also not been explored. A diet rich in fruit and vegetables is associated with a lower risk of acne, which may be attributed in part to the high antioxidant plant polyphenol content of such a diet [26].

Supplementation with omega-3 (2000 mg EPA and DHA) and GLA (400 mg) fatty acids—precursor molecules for prostaglandins and leukotrienes in the inflammatory mediator cascade that tend to tamp down inflammation—resulted in decreased lesion counts in acne patients within 5 weeks [27].

Encouraging increased intake of antioxidants via polyphenol-rich vegetables, and perhaps adding antioxidant supplements (zinc 15–30 mg and preformed vitamin A 1000 IU), carries little risk and is likely to improve impaired antioxidant status for acne patients. High-quality fish oil supplementation at two capsules daily appears to be another reasonable option.

Energy System

Red light penetrates biological tissues and appears to stimulate cytochrome C oxidase, the terminal enzyme of the mitochondrial electron transport chain, resulting in increased ATP production. Oxidized, damaged tissues seem to be more responsive to LILT (low-intensity light treatment) [28]. Clinical application of red light twice daily for 8 weeks showed statistically significant decreases in acne lesion count [29].

Blue light photo-excites the porphyrin produced by *C. acnes*, leading to reactive oxygen species production and bacterial destruction [30]. Clinical trials confirm that this action can decrease acne lesion count [31]. Clinical trials in acne show statistically significant decreases in lesion count after 12 weeks of daily treatment with home-use, combination blue–red LED phototherapy compared with sham light treatment [32].

While the trials are small and vary considerably with regard to frequency and duration of treatment, the risks associated with low-level light exposure are minimal. Theoretical rationale and animal and lab studies, combined with the encouraging clinical reports and high safety profile, make light treatment an attractive addition to the acne and rosacea treatment armamentarium [33–35].

Detoxification System

Yushchenko, the Ukrainian leader poisoned with dioxin in 2004, is a prime example of severe chloracne. Formation of comedones and epidermal cysts around the eyes, in the retroauricular region, and on the scrotum is characteristic [36].

This condition is well described in chemical workers and those with accidental exposure to dioxins used in pesticides, PVC, paper bleaching, and wood preservatives [37]. Dioxins constitute a group of chlorinated dibenzo-*p*-dioxin and dibenzofuran congeners that are largely the by-products of incineration processes and the production of chloro-organic chemicals such as those found in some wood preservatives and herbicides. E-waste is a more recently studied source of exposure [38]. This class of chemicals appears to trigger acne by interfering with vitamin A function [39]. By binding the AhR (aryl hydrocarbon receptor), they upregulate CYP1A1 activity in the sebaceous glands and vessels in the affected skin. This P450 enzyme, one of the primary catabolizers of vitamin A, is not normally expressed in the skin [40]. The blood level of toxicity equivalents that causes chloracne to develop is between 650 and 1200 pg [36].

Given the genetic variability of vitamin A metabolism/catabolism and polymorphism in the AhR and CYPA1A genes, we might reasonably expect some people to be more sensitive than others to the acneigenic potential of dioxins. Both topical and ingested vitamin A can raise levels in the skin and counteract the rapid catabolism of vitamin A that results from dioxin exposure.

Beta-carotene mono-oxidase 1 (BCMO1) converts beta-carotene into two active retinal molecules. Several well-described single nucleotide variants in the BCMO1 gene result in loss of function such that beta-carotene intake results in lower levels of active vitamin A. The combination of two of these alleles has a frequency of 36% in Caucasians [41]. Most multivitamin supplements provide vitamin A as beta-carotene. For our patients with snps in BCMO1 or other vitamin A catabolizing genes, beta-carotene may not provide adequate vitamin A. Perhaps our patients whose acne recurs post isotretinoin require supplementation with preformed vitamin A to compensate for genetic variants in catabolism.

Cardiovascular/Lymphatic Transport System

Rosacea and Flushing

The pathophysiology of rosacea remains incompletely characterized, and, in addition to the proposed mechanisms of innate immune system dysregulation, abnormal responses to commensal organisms, barrier dysfunction, and environmental exposures to UV radiation, there is also a component of neurovascular dysregulation [42]. The effects of this dysregulation are clinically apparent in the rosacea subtypes where flushing, telangiectasia, and erythema are appreciated.

There are both proposed direct and indirect mechanisms for these vascular changes seen in rosacea. One proposed direct mechanism suggests the pathoetiologic role of the neurovascular transient receptor potential vanilloid receptor 1 (TRPV1) which is located on sensory neurons and can be activated by sensory and inflammatory triggers [43, 44]. Patients with rosacea often implicate environmental and dietary triggers with symptoms of cutaneous flushing, and basic science research suggests that the TRPV1 receptors can be activated by heat, dietary triggers, or inflammation, with downstream effects of neurogenic vasodilatation. Secondary mechanisms include UV-mediated changes in dermal structure that promote telangiectasias and flushing, as well as UV-mediated upregulation of VEGF2 that promotes angiogenesis [44]. While not fully understood, the pathogenesis is likely a combinatorial effect of neuroimmune and environmental interactions that result in the heterogeneous inflammatory and vascular phenotypes seen in rosacea subtypes.

Therapeutically, the vascular changes in rosacea can be resistant to the most common anti-inflammatory topical treatments. The FDA has approved a topical alpha-adrenergic agonist (brimonidine) that decreases flushing by direct vasoconstriction of superficial and mid dermal vessels without altering smaller telangiectasias [45]. This topical is most often used as an intermittent treatment to avoid flushing during a specific event, as there have been reports of rebound erythema in the literature. Laser therapies targeting the hemoglobin chromophore remain the mainstay of treatment to reduce unwanted telangiectasias. Topical cover-up strategies with green-tinted makeup have also been employed with success for cosmetic reduction of facial erythema. Finally, trigger avoidance and reduction of UV radiation exposures remain as the mainstays of treatment and active prevention strategies.

Rosacea and Cardiovascular Disease

Motivated by the recent characterization of the cardiovascular disease risk factors for patients with psoriasis, there has been significant interest in evaluating the systemic comorbidities for patients with other common chronic inflammatory conditions [46–48]. Research into the disease associations of rosacea remain in the early stages, and there is conflicting evidence regarding the association of rosacea with gastrointestinal, neurologic, psychiatric, and cardiovascular diseases.

Given the inflammatory and vascular changes noted in many of the rosacea subtypes, there have been multiple recent studies in the dermatologic literature attempting to characterize the cardiovascular disease risk factors for patients with rosacea [49–51]. A 2013 case–control study performed in Turkey demonstrated significantly increased rates of cardiovascular disease risk factors in patients with rosacea compared to matched controls [52]. Another 2015 case–control study performed in Taiwan identified significantly increased rates of dyslipidemia, coronary artery disease, and hypertension in patients with rosacea compared to matched controls [53]. However, several studies have demonstrated no such relationship, and a 2016 Danish case–control study failed to identify any association between rosacea and increased risk of adverse cardiovascular events (myocardial infarction, stroke) or all-cause mortality [54].

In the setting of the conflicting data available to date, specific cardiovascular screening or treatment recommendations are not yet possible. However, in the context of possible etiologic links between neurovascular and immune dysregulation in rosacea, it is reasonable to counsel patients with rosacea to obtain age-appropriate screening and address modifiable risk factors for cardiovascular disease.

Consideration of the potential systemic inflammatory and cardiovascular links to rosacea connects ongoing basic science and epidemiologic research with a holistic assessment of a patient's health. Essentially, this approach strives to create an opportunity for patients motivated to treat their rosacea to simultaneously consider other significant modifiable disease risk factors that may carry benefits beyond their rosacea treatment. The challenge for functional medicine in this area is therefore to identify the subset of patients for whom modification of cardiovascular risk factors also carries a benefit for their cutaneous symptoms.

Hormone/Neurotransmitter Systems

Adult female acne tends to flare with the menses and be distributed in the hormonally sensitive "beard area," and improves in many women using oral contraceptive pills, which hijack ovarian function. Insulin increases 5-alpha reductase activity in the ovary, disrupting ovarian function by increasing conversion of testosterone to the more active dihydrotestosterone [55]. Here again the simple intervention of a low-GL diet can have profound effects on physiology by modulating insulin levels.

Stress is clearly documented as a trigger for acne. Corticotropin-releasing hormone (CRH) is considered the central coordinator for neuroendocrine and behavioral responses to stress. Expression of CRH is increased in the sebaceous glands in acne and stimulates sebum production and steroidogenesis. In keratinocytes, CRH stimulates activity of IL-6 and IL-11, increasing inflammation [56]. A study of diaphragmatic breathing, for 20–30-min sessions over 8 weeks, resulted in decreased cortisol levels in the study group compared with controls [57].

Sleep deprivation raises cortisol [58], which may explain why insufficient sleep is a risk factor for acne in Chinese adolescents [59]. A single night of decreased sleep raises insulin, invoking another mechanism for increased acne [60].

Helping patients understand how sleep and stress directly affect acne can improve compliance with our suggestions for 8 h of nightly uninterrupted sleep and incorporation of breath exercises into their daily routines.

Musculoskeletal System/Cellular Structure

Trans-epidermal water loss is increased in those with acne, reflecting an impaired skin barrier. Given their role in skin barrier function, the decreased ceramides found in those with acne are not surprising [61]. Operating on the assumption that correction of such impairment can contribute to control of acne, minimizing damage by avoiding strong cleansers and applying moisturizers containing ceramides may be helpful. Skin barrier function can be improved by taking flaxseed oil supplementation (four capsules daily) [62]. Animal studies suggest that ingestion of ceramides results in their deposition in the skin [63]. Supplementation with ceramide from konjac (from the plant *Amorphophallus konjac*) improves atopic dermatitis, a disease defined by genetic barrier weakness [64]. Shirataki is a traditional Japanese noodle-like food made from konjac.

Functional Medicine Approach to Treatment of Acne/Rosacea

After gathering information and evaluating the seven clinical imbalances, the clinician and patient decide on which areas to prioritize. A collaborative therapeutic plan is then implemented that blends prescriptions with addressing personalized lifestyle factors. Examples of treatment options that address personalized lifestyle factors include:

- *Sleep and relaxation*
  - Aim for 8 h of uninterrupted sleep nightly.
  - Spend at least a few moments each day doing something that relaxes you.
- *Exercise and movement*
  - Participate in moderate exercise daily to help keep insulin levels lower.
  - Take a few moments to stretch and improve your flexibility each day
- *Nutrition (food, vitamins, minerals, supplements, botanicals, etc.)*
  - Try to consume a nutrient-dense, low-glycemic load diet.
  - Try to include six to nine fist-sized servings of vegetables daily. *Tip*: Aim to eat at least one or two items from each color of the rainbow (red, orange, yellow, green, blue, purple).
  - Minimize added sugars, including sweet beverages.
  - Limit foods made from grain and processed foods (foods that come in a package that are made by a factory vs made by nature).
  - Avoid dairy (except for butter).
  - Consider taking two fish oil capsules daily.

- Consider supplementing with 15–30 mg of zinc in an amino acid chelate form.
- Consider supplementing with preformed vitamin A 1000–5000 IU daily.
- Apply topical niacinamide 2–5% twice daily as a cream or solution.

- *Stress management*
  - Slow and deepen the breath several times daily. Cell phone applications can be useful.
- *Relationships and community connections*
  - Connect with your family, friends, and co-workers.
  - Get involved with local community volunteer programs.
- *Environmental factors (quality of air, water, skin care products, etc.)*
  - For postauricular acne, consider sensitivity to dioxins.
  - Organically grown foods help decrease exposure to dioxins from pesticides.
  - Consider vitamin A supplementation to compensate for rapid catabolism induced by dioxins.
- *Mental factors (cognition, perception, and psychosocial factors)*
  - Functional medicine empowers the patient by including them in the planning of their program. Much of the action plan lies directly in their hands.
  - Collaborate with a therapist or psychologist to help mindset and seeing a different perspective.
- *Emotional factors (awareness and regulation of emotions)*
  - Explore resources to learn about emotions and how to manage them.
  - Figure out what gives you joy and add in those activities that bring you joy at least once daily.
  - If not managed with stress management, consider counseling/therapy.

- *Spiritual connections (sense of purpose and meaning)*
  - Explore the depth of your life purpose using resources that connect with a belief system that resonates with you.

The lifestyle changes addressed are individualized based on the assessment of the patient's clinical imbalances and goals and priorities set collaboratively by the patient and clinician. Partnerships with other practitioners and clinicians such as psychologist, acupuncturist, mind/body specialist, nutritionist, health coach, subspecialty physicians, etc. is commonly integrated into the therapeutic plan to adequately address lifestyle factors.

Conclusion

The functional medicine approach to acne and rosacea is a comprehensive methodology to unveil core clinical imbalances. A collaborative, individualized treatment plan is based on goals and priorities determined by the patient and clinician. Therapeutic treatment plans include implementing lifestyle changes, partnership with other practitioners, as well as prescription treatment options.

References

1. National Rosacea Society. Rosacea dairy booklet. [Online] Available at: https://www.rosacea.org/patients/materials/rosacea-diary-booklet
2. American Academy of Dermatology. Available at: aad.org/public. Accessed 2011.
3. Fulton JE, Plewig G, Kligman AM. Effect of chocolate on acne vulgaris. JAMA. 1969;210(11):2071–4.
4. Anderson PC. Food as the cause of acne. Am Fam Physician. 1971;3:102–3.
5. Juhl CR, Bergholdt HKM, Miller IM, Jemec GBE, Kanters JK, Ellervik C. Dairy intake and acne vulgaris: a systematic review and meta-analysis of 78,529 children, adolescents, and young adults. Nutrients. 2018;10(8):1049.

6. Barbieri JS, Spaccarelli N, Margolis DJ, James WD. Approaches to limit systemic antibiotic use in acne: systemic alternatives, emerging topical therapies, dietary modification, and laser and light-based treatments. J Am Acad Dermatol. 2019;80(2):538–49.
7. Melnik B. Linking diet to acne metabolomics, inflammation and comedogenesis. An update. Clin Cosmet Investig Dermatol. 2015;8:371–88.
8. Agamia NF, Abdallah DM, Sorour O, Mourad B, Younan DN. Skin expression of mammalian target of rapamycin and forkhead box transcription factor 01, and serum insulin-like growth factor-1 in patients with acne vulgaris and their relationship with diet. Br J Dermatol. 2016;174:1299–307.
9. Moran A, Jacobs DR, Steinberger J, Hong CP, Prineas R, Luepker R, et al. Insulin resistance during puberty: results from clamp studies in 357 children. Diabetes. 1999;48(10):2039–44.
10. Schmitt JV, Masuda PY, Miot HA. Acne in women: clinical patterns in different age-groups. An Bras Dermatol. 2009;84:349–54.
11. Jenkins DJA, Kendall CWC, Augustin LSA, et al. Glycemic index: overview of implications in health and disease. Am J Clin Nutr. 2002;76:226S–73S.
12. Kaufman WH. The diet and acne. Arch Dermatol. 1983;119:276.
13. Anderson JW, O'Neal DS, Riddell-Mason S, Floore TL, Dillon DW, Oeltgen PR. Postprandial serum glucose, insulin and lipoprotein responses to high- and low-fiber diets. Metabolism. 1995;44(7):848–54.
14. Hoyt G, Hickey MS, Cordain L. Dissociation of the glycaemic and insulinaemic responses to whole and skimmed milk. Br J Nutr. 2005;93(2):175–7.
15. Heaney RP, McCarron DA, Dawson-Hughes B, Oparil S, Berga SL, Stern JS, et al. Dietary changes favorably affect bone remodeling in older adults. J Am Diet Assoc. 1999;99(10):1228–33.
16. Ben-Amital D, Laron Z. Effect of insulin-like growth factor-1 deficiency or administration on the occurrence of acne. J Eur Acad Dermatol Venereol. 2011;25(8):950–4.
17. Parodi A, Paolino S, Greco A, Drago F, Mansi C, Rebora A, et al. Small intestinal bacterial overgrowth in rosacea: clinical effectiveness of its eradication. Clin Gastroenterol Hepatol. 2008;6:759–64.
18. Chedid V, Dhalla S, Clarke JO, Roland BC, Dunbar KB, Koh J, et al. Herbal therapy is equivalent to rifaximin for the treatment of small intestinal bacterial overgrowth. Glob Adv Health Med. 2014;3(3):16–24.

19. Salem I, Ramser A, Isham N, Ghannoum MA. The gut microbiome as a major regulator of the gut-skin axis. Front Microbiol. 2018;9:1459.
20. Melnik B. Acne and genetics. In: Zouboulis CC, Christos C, Katsambas AD, Kligman AM, editors. Pathogenesis and treatment of acne and rosacea. Berlin: Springer-Verlag; 2014. p. 109–30.
21. Block ML, Zecca L, Hong JS. Microglia-medicated neurotoxicity: uncovering the molecular mechanisms. Nat Rev Neurosci. 2007;8:57–69.
22. Arican O, Kurutas EB, Sasmaz S. Oxidative stress in patients with acne vulgaris. Mediat Inflamm. 2005;2005(6):380–4.
23. Abdel FNS, Shaheen MA, Ebrahim AA, El Okda ES. Tissue and blood superoxide dismutase activities and malondialdehyde levels in different clinical severities of acne vulgaris. Br J Dermatol. 2008;159(5):1086–91.
24. Amer M, Bahgat MR, Tosson Z, Abdel Mowla MY, Amer K. Serum zinc in acne vulgaris. Int J Dermatol. 1982;21(8):481–4.
25. Labadarios D, Cilliers J, Visser L, Van Stuijvenberg ME, Shephard GS, Wium D, et al. Vitamin A in acne vulgaris. Exp Dermatol. 1987;12(6):432–6.
26. Di Landro A, Cazzaniga S, Cusano F, Bonci A, Carla C, Musumeci ML, et al. Adult female acne and associated risk factors: results of a multicenter case-control study in Italy. J Am Acad Dermatol. 2016;75(6):1134–41.
27. Jung JY, Kwon HH, Hong JS, Yoon JY, Park MS, Jang MY, et al. Effect of dietary supplementation with Omega-3 fatty acid and gamma-linolenic acid on acne vulgaris: a randomised, double blind, controlled trial. Acta Derm Venereol. 2014;94(5):521–5.
28. Tafur J, Mills PJ. Low-intensity light therapy: exploring the role of redox mechanisms. Photomed Laser Surg. 2008;26(4):323–8.
29. Na JI, Suh DH. Red light phototherapy alone is effective for acne vulgaris: randomized, single-blinded clinical trial. Dermatol Surg. 2007;33:1228–33.
30. Arakane K, Ryu A, Hayashi C. Singlet oxygen (1 delta g) generation from coproporphyrin in Propionibacterium acnes on irradiation. Biochem Biophys Res Commun. 1996;223:578–82.
31. Tzung TY, Wu KH, Huang ML. Blue light phototherapy in the treatment of acne. Photodermatol Photoimmunol Photomed. 2004;20:266–9.
32. Kwon HH, Lee JB, Yoon JY, Park SY, Ryu HH, Park BM, et al. The clinical and histological effect of home-use, combination

blue-red LED phototherapy for mild-to-moderate acne vulgaris in Korean patients: a double-blind, randomized controlled trial. Br J Dermatol. 2013;168(5):1088–94.

33. Papageorgiou P, Katsambas A, Chu A. Phototherapy with blue (415 nm) and red (660 nm) light in the treatment of acne vulgaris. Br J Dermatol. 2000;142:973–8.
34. Goldberg DJ, Russell BA. Combination blue (415 nm) and red (633 nm) LED phototherapy in the treatment of mild to severe acne vulgaris. J Cosmet Laser Ther. 2006;8:71–5.
35. Lee SY, You CE, Park MY. Blue and red light combination LED phototherapy for acne vulgaris in patients with skin phototype IV. Lasers Surg Med. 2007;39:180–8.
36. Coenraads PJ, Olie K, Tang NJ. Blood lipid concentrations of dioxins and dibenzofurans causing chloracne. Br J Dermatol. 1999;141:694–7.
37. Bond GG, McLaren EA, Brenner FE, Cook RR. Incidence of chloracne among chemical workers potentially exposed to chlorinated dioxins. J Occup Med. 1989;31:771–4.
38. Ma J, Kannan K, Cheng J, Horii Y, Wu Q, Wang W. Concentrations, profiles, and estimated human exposures for polychlorinated dibenzo-p-dioxins and dibenzofurans from electronic waste recycling facilities and a chemical industrial complex in Eastern China. Environ Sci Technol. 2008;42(22):8252–9.
39. Coenraads PJ, Brouwer A, Olie K, Tang N. Chloracne. Some recent issues. Dermatol Clin. 1994;12(3):569–76.
40. Fabbrocini G, Kaya G, Caseiro Silverio P, De Vita V, Kaya A, Fontao F, et al. Aryl hydrocarbon receptor activation in acne vulgaris skin: a case series from the region of Naples, Italy. Dermatology. 2015;231:334–8.
41. Kim YJ, Moon SM, Yang YJ, et al. Single nucleotide polymorphisms in the β-carotene 15,15-monooxygenase coding gene and health outcomes in Korean adults. FASEB. 2012;26:824–13.
42. Two AM, Wu W, Gallo RL, Hata TR. Rosacea: part I. Introduction, categorization, histology, pathogenesis, and risk factors. J Am Acad Dermatol. 2015;72(5):749–58; quiz 759–60.
43. Holmes AD, Spoendlin J, Chien AL, Baldwin H, Chang ALS. Evidence-based update on rosacea comorbidities and their common physiologic pathways. J Am Acad Dermatol. 2018;78(1):156–66.
44. Steinhoff M, Buddenkotte J, Aubert J, Sulk M, Novak P, Schwab VD, et al. Clinical, cellular, and molecular aspects in the

pathophysiology of rosacea. J Investig Dermatol Symp Proc. 2011;15(1):2–11.
45. Two AM, Wu W, Gallo RL, Hata TR. Rosacea: part II. Topical and systemic therapies in the treatment of rosacea. J Am Acad Dermatol. 2015;72(5):761–70; quiz 771–2.
46. Rainer BM, Fischer AH, Luz Felipe da Silva D, Kang S, Chien AL. Rosacea is associated with chronic systemic diseases in a skin severity–dependent manner: results of a case-control study. J Am Acad Dermatol. 2015;73(4):604–8.
47. Haber R, El Gemayel M. Comorbidities in rosacea: a systematic review and update. J Am Acad Dermatol. 2018;78(4):786–792.e8.
48. Aldrich N, Gerstenblith M, Fu P, Tuttle MS, Varma P, Gotow E, et al. Genetic vs environmental factors that correlate with rosacea: a cohort-based survey of twins. JAMA Dermatol. 2015;151(11):1213–9.
49. Dosal JR, Rodriguez GL, Pezon CF, Li H, Keri JE. Effect of tetracyclines on the development of vascular disease in veterans with acne or rosacea: a retrospective cohort study. J Invest Dermatol. 2014;134(8):2267–9.
50. Dosal J, Keri J. Rosacea and cardiovascular disease: is there an association? J Am Acad Dermatol. 2015;73(2):308–9.
51. Marshall VD, Moustafa F, Hawkins SD, Balkrishnan R, Feldman SR. Cardiovascular disease outcomes associated with three major inflammatory dermatologic diseases: a propensity-matched case control study. Dermatol Ther. 2016;6(4):649–58.
52. Duman N, Ersoy Evans S, Atakan N. Rosacea and cardiovascular risk factors: a case control study. J Eur Acad Dermatol Venereol. 2014;28(9):1165–9.
53. Hua TC, Chung PI, Chen YJ, Wu LC, Chen YD, Hwang CY, et al. Cardiovascular comorbidities in patients with rosacea: a nationwide case-control study from Taiwan. J Am Acad Dermatol. 2015;73(2):249–54.
54. Egeberg A, Hansen PR, Gislason GH, Thyssen JP. Assessment of the risk of cardiovascular disease in patients with rosacea. J Am Acad Dermatol. 2016;75(2):336–9.
55. Kayampilly PP, Wanamaker BL, Stewart JA, Wagner CL, Menon KM. Stimulatory effect of insulin on 5α-reductase type 1 (SRD5A1) expression through an akt-dependent pathway in ovarian granulosa cells. Endocrinology. 2010;151(10):5030–7.
56. Ganceviciene R, Graziene V, Fimmel S, Zouboulis CC. Involvement of the corticotropin-releasing hormone system in the pathogenesis of acne vulgaris. Br J Dermatol. 2009;160:345–52.

57. Ma X, Yue ZQ, Gong ZQ, Zhang H, Duan NY, Shi YT, et al. The effect of diaphragmatic breathing on attention, negative affect and stress in healthy adults. Front Psychol. 2017;8:874.
58. Leproult R, Copinschi G, Buxton O, Van Cauter E. Sleep loss results in an elevation of cortisol levels the next morning. Sleep. 1997;20:865–70.
59. Wu TQ, Mei SQ, Zhang JX, Gong LF, Wu FJ, Wu WH, et al. Prevalence and risk factors of facial acne vulgaris among Chinese adolescents. Int J Adolesc Med Health. 2007;19(4):407–12.
60. Donga E, van Dijk M, van Dijk JG, Biermasz NR, Lammers GJ, van Kralingen KW, et al. A single night of partial sleep deprivation induces insulin resistance in multiple pathways in healthy subjects. J Clin Endocrinol Metab. 2010;95(6):2963–8.
61. Pappas A, Kendall AC, Brownbridge LC, Batchvarova N, Nicolaou A. Seasonal changes in epidermal ceramides are linked to impaired barrier function in acne patients. Exp Dermatol. 2018;27:833–6.
62. Neukam K, De Spirt S, Stahl W, Bejot M, Maurette JM, Tronnier H, et al. Supplementation of flaxseed oil diminishes skin sensitivity and improves skin barrier function and condition. Skin Pharmacol Physiol. 2011;24(2):67–74.
63. Ueda O, Hasegawa M, Kitamura S. Distribution in skin of ceramide after oral aministration to rats. Drug Metab Pharmacokinet. 2009;24(2):180–4.
64. Kimata H. Improvement of atopic dermatitis and reduction of skin allergic responses by oral intake of konjac ceramide. Pediatr Dermatol. 2006;23:386–9.

Chapter 10
Ayurvedic Approaches to Acne and Rosacea

Aunna Pourang and Raja K. Sivamani

Introduction

Ayurveda, meaning "knowledge of life" in Sanskrit, is a traditional form of medicine that originated in India and is thought to be between 5000 and 15,000 years old. Ayurvedic medicine is built upon the principles that are meant to describe the human body in terms of balance vs imbalance. Diagnostic descriptions are heavily focused on understanding how the body may be shifting out of balance, and interventions are aimed to restore balance. Imbalances encompass physical, psychological, emotional, and spiritual states.

Ayurvedic Building Blocks

The Role of Elements

The human body is thought to consist of elements that make up the universe: earth, water, fire, air, and space. These words are translated from the Sanskrit origins and lose their meaning when put in context of the English words, but suffice it to

---

A. Pourang · R. K. Sivamani (✉)
Department of Dermatology, University of California – Davis, Sacramento, CA, USA

R. N. Rupani, P. A. Lio (eds.), *Integrative Dermatology*,
https://doi.org/10.1007/978-3-030-58954-7_10

say that the elements serve both a literal and metaphorical interpretation. Please see Table 10.1 for how each of the elements is represented broadly and how it specifically relates to the skin.

Of special note is the concept of ether, as this is the most abstract yet the most physically present. Ether represents the space that is occupied by other things like structure, fluid, cells, etc. With aging, there is a loss of tissue and thickness of collagen. This can be thought of as an increase in ether, as the potential space now takes up more space than the actual skin tissue.

The Role of Doshas

Various combinations of these elements give rise to the three *doshas* (biological energies), seven *dhatus* (tissues), and three

Table 10.1 Ayurvedic elements and their relation to biochemistry and the skin

Element	Broad representation	Biochemical/ physical representation	Representation in the skin
Earth	Structure and form	Molecular structure	Collagen and skin structure
Water	Fluids and absorption	Heat capacity and fluids	Sebum, skin hydration, antioxidants
Fire	Transformation and heat	Enzymatic reactions and inflammation	Redness, inflammation
Air	Motion	Cell division, blood flow, transmission of signals/ hormones	Viscoelasticity of the skin, scaling when cell division is too fast
Ether/ space	Potential space	Physical space	Physical space

TABLE 10.2 Doshas in Ayurveda

Doshas	Compositional elements	Overall function in healthy skin	General symptoms when imbalanced
Vata	Air and ether	Elasticity, normal cell division	Dryness, scaling, thin skin
Pitta	Fire and water	Normal metabolism	Inflammation
Kapha	Earth and water	Normal structure of collagen and appendages	Edema, fibrosis, oiliness

malas (waste products). The three biological energies or doshas are the more commonly discussed concepts in Ayurveda (Table 10.2).

Ayurveda is typically thought of as a balance vs imbalance in the doshas. When thinking about these doshas, it's important to note that Ayurveda describes two different states for the body: the balanced state and the current imbalance.

Prakriti Versus Vikriti: Natural Constitution Versus Imbalances

The balanced state is also known as the natural constitution or the *prakriti*. It is thought that each person is born with a natural balanced constitution called prakriti and that through external factors such as a poor diet and stress, one can develop an imbalanced state, known as *vikriti*. Prakriti relates to the tendency toward certain imbalances, such as the tendency toward oily skin and acne, the tendency toward dry skin, or the tendency toward skin sensitivity. Support for the use of a prakriti system has been supported by rigorous genomic association studies that have clustered genotype with the Ayurvedic prakriti typing [1].

As opposed to the prakriti, imbalances are known as vikriti. Imblances lead to the presence of symptoms and disease. Imbalances and illnesses are diagnosed by history and exam. Treatment of diseases is tailored to suit an individual based on the vikriti or imbalances [2]. Regardless of the prakriti, which relates to constitution and tendencies, vikriti relates to true imbalances that develop and may lead to symptoms. In Ayurveda, interventions are directed toward addressing the vikriti. Many of the interventions that are recommended to bring one back into balance involve proper diet, lifestyle, and herbal remedies. One of the main tenets of Ayurvedic philosophy revolves around optimal digestion.

While the Ayurvedic ideology is different from modern medicine, it has several relatable factors with Western medicine. The prakriti may relate to genetic predispositions. As we now understand, epigenetic influences and our lifestyle can serve a role in how those genetic predispositions manifest, much like how prakriti relates to tendencies, but our actions and habits are what drive whether those tendencies manifest into true imbalances. Similarly, symptoms relate to Ayurvedic vikriti, and reduction of the imbalances described by the vikriti relates to the concept of treating symptoms. The additional feature of vikriti treatment is an understanding that the treatment frequently requires a shift in habits, diets, and lifestyle rather than engaging in any one modality (Table 10.3).

The doshas can be further subtyped into subdoshas, but this is beyond the scope of this chapter. For those motivated, more information can be found elsewhere [3].

TABLE 10.3 Vikriti with the imbalances in the doshas

Doshas	**Examples of presentation**
Vata	Dry skin Thin skin Atrophic
Pitta	Inflamed skin Redness
Kapha	Oily skin Thickened

Skin Disease in Ayurveda: Acne as a Model

Kushta is a word used to describe skin diseases. Based on the description of these diseases in ancient Ayurvedic texts, modern correlations of dermatologic diseases have been postulated. This chapter will focus on acne as an illustrative example of how a skin disease is approached in Ayurveda.

In Ayurveda, acne vulgaris has been referred to as *Mukhadushika* (one which disfigures the face) and *Yavanpidika* (eruptions occurring on the face during adolescence) [4–7]. The Ayurvedic explanation for the pathophysiology of acne is thought to arise as a result of an increase in *pitta*, causing inflammation, and increase in *kapha*, causing increased oil formation [6]. The modern correlate for pitta imbalances can be likened to inflammatory mediators and toxins, such as interleukin-1and LPS, respectively, which have been found to be elevated in the serum of patients with acne [8, 9].

In Ayurveda, acne is thought to be caused by intake of fried and unhealthy foods, meat, dairy, improper food combinations, alcohol, stress, hormonal imbalances, and an exposure to moist temperate climates [10–13]. Some of these ancient concepts have been demonstrated scientifically as dairy, high-glycemic index foods, stress, hot humid climate, and hormonal imbalances—all have been associated with acne [14–18].

Ayurvedic tradition still has a strong influence in India, as patients with acne perceive the importance of diet and dietary changes in modulating skin disease when compared to those without skin disease [13].

Treating Acne Using an Ayurvedic Approach

The overall goal is to reduce and address the imbalances that are associated with acne. The doshas that tend to be out of balance are pitta and kapha, although there are many variations in the imbalances depending on symptoms in the skin, digestion, and psychology. There are several ways to treat acne using Ayurveda, from lifestyle modifications to oral supplements, intranasal administration of herbs, and topical applications of *lepa* (paste) or *taila* (oil).

Lifestyle Modification: Stress Management and Proper Diet

In general, Ayurveda strongly promotes lifestyle modification. Meditation to help decrease stress and a tailored diet may be recommended as part of a treatment plan. Diets are tailored to the individual's imbalances, but overall, a whole food plant-based diet rich in fresh greens is recommended and avoiding triggers, such as spicy, oily, and fried foods [19].

Ayurvedic Oral and Topical Treatments of Acne

Mugdha rasa is a specialized oral formulation used to treat acne. It usually contains *Rubia cordifolia*, *Hemidesmus indicus*, *Azadirachta indica*, and *Curcuma longa.* While formulations in Ayurveda typically consist of multiple herbs, they are used with a certain intent [20–22]. In this case, these herbs all help balance pitta and kapha imbalances, which are found in those with acne. In vitro, when these compounds were exposed to polymorphonuclear neutrophils (PMNs) isolated from the peripheral blood of healthy volunteers, a statistically significant suppression of reactive oxygen species (ROS) induced by *C. acnes* culture supernatant was noted [23, 24]. These herbs also suppressed *C. acnes*-induced TNF-α and IL-8 production [23]. Notably, there need to be more clinical studies with Ayurvedic subtyping to better assess the efficacy of these formulations in acne and in the Ayurvedic subtyping system.

A non-randomized clinical trial using oral *Varnya Mahakashaya* and a topical formulation called *chandra prabha lepa*, containing *Brassica campestris* (field mustard), *Acorus calamus* (calamus or sweet flag), *Symplocos racemo-*

sus (lodhra), *Buchanania lanzan* (chironji), *Lens culinaris* (lentils), and sodium chloride improved acne [25]. *Lepa* pastes are often used for their astringent and anti-inflammatory properties [11].

A clinical trial using an intervention of oral formulation containing *Picrorhiza kurroa* (kutki), *Andrographis paniculata* (green chiretta), *Eclipta alba* (false daisy), *Tinospora cordifolia* (guduchi), *Saussurea lappa* (kuth), *Embelia ribes* (vidanga or false black pepper), *Curcuma longa* (turmeric), *Azadirachta indica* (neem), *Cassia fistula* (Indian laburnum), and *Psoralea corylifolia* (babchi), along with a topical formulation containing *Aloe barbadensis* (aloe vera), *Alternanthera sessilis* (*ponnanganni*), and *Rubia cordifolia* (Indian mader or manjistha), showed improvement in patients with grade II and III acne, without serious adverse reactions [26]. The more validated measures of lesions counts were not assessed in this study.

In a double-blinded trial, an oral formulation containing the bitter herbs *Holarrhena antidysenterica* (kutaj), *Emblica officinalis* (amalaki), *Embelia ribes* (vidanga), and *Zingiber officinale* (ginger) showed a significant improvement in inflammatory and noninflammatory lesions compared with baseline or placebo [27]. The formulation was designed to balance pitta and kapha, but the study was underpowered in several of the treatment groups. However, the findings warrant expanded studies.

A phase 2 clinical trial was conducted using oral Ayurvedic preparations with or without the use of topical Ayurvedic formulations containing *Aloe barbadensis* (aloe vera), *Azadirachta indica* (neem), *Curcuma longa* (turmeric), *Hemidesmus indicus* (Indian sarsaparilla), *Terminalia chebula* (chebulic myrobalan), *Terminalia arjuna* (arjun), and *Withania somnifera* (ashwagandha) [7]. *Piper longum* (long pepper) extract was added to improve the bioavailability of the oral preparation. The combined treatment of oral and topical formulation showed better results than the tablets alone when compared to placebo [7]. This study was limited by the lack of lesion counts as a study measure, and some of the treatment groups were largely underpowered, with the true placebo group consisting of only one subject.

A popular bitter herb used in Ayurveda, *Commiphora mukul* (guggul), reduced inflammatory lesions of nodulocystic acne in a double-blinded clinical trial when compared to tetracycline [28]. Another study demonstrated an improvement of moderate and severe acne when treated with *Commiphora mukul* [29]. It has been suggested that the antilipolytic activity of *Commiphora mukul* reduces sebum secretion, thus inhibiting triglyceride lipolysis by bacterial lipases to free fatty acids, which promote acne formation [28–31]. From an Ayurvedic perspective, this relates to kapha balancing properties. A topical formulation of *Commiphora mukul* was found to have anti-inflammatory activity [32]. *Commiphora mukul* also has antioxidant capabilities [33].

An anti-acne topical gel formulation made with tea tree oil, aloe vera gel, and extracts of *Ocimum sanctum* and *Tabernaemontana divaricata* showed inhibitory activity toward *C. acnes*, though not as much as tetracycline. The aloe vera gel and tea tree oil tested alone did not have significant activity toward *C. acnes* [34].

AHPL/AYTOP/0213 cream (Ari Healthcare Private Ltd., India) is a polyherbal formulation developed to treat acne vulgaris, hyperpigmentation, and various skin disorders. It contains *Berberis aristata* (daruharidra), *Symplocos racemosa* (lodhra), *Glycyrrhiza glabra* (licorice), *Myristica fragrans* (jatiphala), *Rubia cordifolia* (manjistha), *Acorus calamus* (vacha), *Coriandrum sativum* (dhanyaka), and *Salmalia malabarica* (shalami). This cream showed antimicrobial activity against *P. acnes*, *S. epidermidis*, and *S. aureus*, comparable to clindamycin [35].

An in vitro study comparing the inhibitory effects of creams containing various amounts of flavonoids or tannins from *Terminalia arjuna* showed all developed formulations had inhibitory effect on *C. acnes* and *S. epidermidis*. The formulation, containing 2% flavonoid fraction, had stronger inhibitory activity than that of other developed formulations [36].

Proposed Mechanisms of Action for Ayurvedic Treatments of Acne

Most of the Ayurvedic herbs mentioned in the studies above are considered to be bitter, and the formulations have kapha and pitta balancing properties. They are also recommended by Ayurvedic practitioners due to their ability to stimulate *agni* (gastric fire) [37]. Bitter herbs have, in fact, been shown to both stimulate gastric secretion and digestion and improve acne [37, 38]. Hypochlorhydria has been associated with acne and rosacea and is also thought to cause intestinal dysbiosis, which is also thought to play a role in these diseases [39–43].

Other bitter, berberine-containing herbs such as *Berberis vulgaris* (barberry) and *Mahonia aquifolium* (Oregon grape) contain alkaloids that have antimicrobial and anti-inflammatory activity [44, 45]. Berberine has been shown to inhibit abnormal lipogenesis in the sebaceous glands of hamsters, and Oregon grape extracts have demonstrated activity against *C. acnes* in vitro [45, 46].

The gut microbiome is gaining evidence and support as a mediator of inflammation in the body and may also play a role in acne [42, 47]. A low-glycemic load diet, rich in plant fibers and low in processed foods, has been associated with an improvement in acne through various proposed mechanisms. The gut dysbiosis theory postulates that since patients with acne have been found to have gut dysbiosis, restoring gut microbiome homeostasis may help improve acne [48]. Just as oral probiotics have been shown to mediate inflammation in skin disease and topical probiotics can improve acne, plants and herbs may also have similar therapeutic potential [49–52]. Herbs and plant-based foods rich in fiber and polyphenols can also act like prebiotics and interact with the gut microbiome, altering microbial metabolites such as short-chain fatty acids (SCFAs) and lipopolysaccharides (LPS), which are involved in acne pathogenesis [9, 53, 54].

In Ayurveda, high-glycemic diets aggravate kapha imbalances, while low-glycemic diets counter imbalances in pitta and kapha. Acne has not only been associated with a high-glycemic load diet, but low-glycemic load diets have been associated with an improvement in acne [55–57]. Hyperinsulinemia, as a result of high-glycemic load foods, increases serum levels of insulin-like growth factor-1 and reduces serum levels of insulin-like growth factor binding protein-3 and, in turn, is thought to increase keratinocyte proliferation and stimulate hormone production [58–60]. Moreover, gut dysbiosis has also been associated with insulin resistance [61]. Prebiotic compounds found in plants, such as resistant starches, insoluble fiber, and fructooligosaccharides, have been correlated with greater insulin sensitivity and less inflammation [62–64]. Furthermore, herbs like berberine and guggul may also improve insulin sensitivity [65, 66].

Secondary metabolites of plants such as alkaloids, flavonoids, tannins, and other polyphenols are thought to confer antioxidant, antimicrobial, and anti-inflammatory properties, which may also be responsible for their effectiveness in treating acne [67, 68]. Many of these effects also apply to topical therapy as well. See Table 10.4 for Ayurvedic herbs and the likely anti-acne properties they possess.

Table 10.4 Ayurvedic herbs and their potential anti-acne properties

Herb name	Effect on Ayurvedic doshas	Potential anti-acne properties
Aloe barbadensis		Has topical anti-inflammatory activity equivalent to hydrocortisone [69] Contains salicylic acid [70]
Azadirachta indica (neem)		Antibacterial toward *C. acnes* [71] Suppresses reactive oxygen species (ROS), TNF-α and IL-8 induced by *C. acnes* [23]
Berberis vulgaris (barberry)		Inhibits abnormal lipogenesis the sebaceous glands of hamsters [46] Improves insulin sensitivity [65]
Commiphora mukul (guggul)		Antilipolytic [30] Anti-inflammatory activity [32] Antioxidant capabilities [33] Improves insulin sensitivity [66]
Coscinium fenestratum		Inhibits *C. acnes* [72]
Cucurbita pepo		Inhibits *C. acnes* [72]

(continued)

Table 10.4 (continued)

Herb name	Effect on Ayurvedic doshas	Potential anti-acne properties
Curcuma longa (turmeric)		Inhibits the growth of *Staphylococcus epidermidis* and *Staphylococcus aureus* [73, 74] Photoactivated curcumin inhibits the growth of *C. acnes* [75] Suppresses reactive oxygen species (ROS), TNF-α and IL-8 induced by *C. acnes* [23]
Eclipta alba		Inhibits *C. acnes* [72]
Embelia ribes (Vidanga)		Inhibits *C. acnes* and *S. epidermidis* [76, 77]
Emblica officinalis (amalaki)		Acts as an antioxidant [78] Broad spectrum antibacterial activity [79]
Euphorbia hirta		Inhibits *C. acnes* [72]
Hemidesmus indicus		Inhibits *C. acnes* [72] Anti-inflammatory and antioxidant capabilities, in addition to containing a high terpenoid content, the latter of which have also been found to have antibacterial activity against *C. acnes* [72, 80, 81] Suppresses reactive oxygen species (ROS), induced TNF-α and IL-8 induced by *C. acnes* [23] Broad-spectrum antibacterial activity [79]

Holarrhena antidysenterica (kutaj)	Broad spectrum antibacterial activity [79, 82]
Glycyrrhiza glabra (licorice)	Inhibits growth of *C. acnes in vitro* but is not associated with bacterial resistance [83]
Piper longum (long pepper)	Antioxidant and antimicrobial properties [84]
Rubia cordifolia	Suppresses reactive oxygen species (ROS), induced TNF-α and IL-8 induced by *C. acnes* [23]
Symplocos racemosa	Strong inhibitory effects toward *C. acnes* and *S. epidermidis* in vitro, thought to be related to its relatively high alkaloid content [72]
Tephrosia purpurea	Inhibits *C. acnes* [72]
Terminalia arjuna	Inhibitory effect of flavonoid and tannins on the *C. acnes* and *S. epidermidis* [36]
Terminalia chebula	Inhibition of *C. acnes* lipase [85]
Tinospora cordifolia	Antioxidant and antimicrobial properties [84] Immunopotentiator [86]

Conclusion

Ancient Ayurvedic wisdom is relevant today, as the central tenets include a holistic approach that depends upon modification of diet, stress, and use of oral and topical herbs. Medications can be used alongside Ayurveda, which allows for a true integrative approach. Using acne as an example, we have illustrated how acne can be addressed from an Ayurvedic perspective.

The increased prevalence of acne in modern times is thought to be multifactorial and is likely related to unhealthy diet and high stress, which can alter the gut microbiome [87, 88]. Many of the medications used to treat acne cause side effects, such as skin irritation (retinoids) and antibiotic resistance (antibiotics), the latter of which has been seen increasingly with *C. acnes* and *S. epidermidis* [89, 90].

Many Ayurvedic herbal formulations have been shown to have decreased antimicrobial resistance and are generally well tolerated. Since polyphenols have been found to act synergistically with various antibiotics against multidrug-resistant microorganisms, it is worth investigating this potential of plant compounds in human studies [67, 79].

Many of the scientific investigations for the Ayurvedic treatment of acne lack power or do not used standardized and validated assessment outcomes [22, 91]. Another limitation is that the enrolled subjects are not subtyped based on their Ayurvedic vikriti, and this limits the evidence to simply the Western model of acne instead of taking the Ayurvedic diagnosis into account as well. High-quality randomized, controlled clinical trials are necessary to continue to investigate the benefits of various Ayurvedic treatments for acne vulgaris and to subtype the effects based on the Ayurvedic vikriti along with the Western diagnosis.

Finally, it is important to note that some Ayurvedic supplements have been found to have high levels of heavy metals in them. However, many reputable companies do exist which produce high-quality products and test for contaminants such as heavy metals and bacterial contamination. Future high-quality studies will depend on collaboration between well-trained researchers and high-quality sources of herbs to drive well-designed studies in this area.

References

1. Govindaraj P, Nizamuddin S, Sharath A, Jyothi V, Rotti H, Raval R, et al. Genome-wide analysis correlates Ayurveda Prakriti. Sci Rep. 2015;5:15786.
2. Routh HB, Bhowmik KR. Traditional Indian medicine in dermatology. Clin Dermatol. 1999;17(1):41–7.
3. Lad V. Textbook of Ayurveda, Vol. 1: Fundamental principles of Ayurveda. Albaquerque: The Ayurvedic Press; 2002.
4. Shukla R, Verma AS. Concept of Kshudraroga in Brihattrayi and Laghuttrayi. J AYUSH. 2014;3:14–23.
5. Singh S, Byadgi PS, Rai NP. Concept of dermatological disorders in Ayurveda. Int J Ayurvedic Herb Med. 2015;5(4):1964–75.
6. Chowdhury K, Dhakar R, Patil SB, Jain R, Datta N. Role of Rohitaka and Sharapunkha on Mukhadushika. Int J Ayurvedic Herb Med. 2013;3:1159–72.
7. Lalla JK, Nandedkar SY, Paranjape MH, Talreja NB. Clinical trials of ayurvedic formulations in the treatment of acne vulgaris. J Ethnopharmacol. 2001;78(1):99–102.
8. Tanghetti EA. The role of inflammation in the pathology of acne. J Clin Aesthet Dermatol. 2013;6(9):27–35.
9. Juhlin L, Michaelsson G. Fibrin microclot formation in patients with acne. Acta Derm Venereol. 1983;63(6):538–40.
10. Kumar V, Khatri S, Meena KL. A view over Yuvana Pidika with special reference to acne. Int J Ayu Pharm Chem. 2017;6(1):61–9.
11. Upasani SA, Nipanikar SU. Review on Yuvanpidika vis-a-vis acne vulgaris. Int J Pharm Pharm Res. 2016;5(3):77–94.
12. Gaur G, Pal S, Kulratan. Yuvnan Pidika – a conceptual study W.S.R. acne vulgaris. Ayushdhara. 2018;5(1):1564–8.
13. Kulkarni M, Keny D, Potey AV, Tripathi RK. A cross-sectional study to assess the incompatible dietary behavior of patients suffering from skin diseases: a pilot study. J Ayurveda Integr Med. 2016;7(2):113–8.
14. Juhl CR, Bergholdt HKM, Miller IM, Jemec GBE, Kanters JK, Ellervik C. Dairy intake and acne vulgaris: a systematic review and meta-analysis of 78,529 children, adolescents, and young adults. Nutrients. 2018;10(8):1049.

15. Costa A, Lage D, Moises TA. Acne and diet: truth or myth? An Bras Dermatol. 2010;85(3):346–53.
16. Zari S, Alrahmani D. The association between stress and acne among female medical students in Jeddah, Saudi Arabia. Clin Cosmet Investig Dermatol. 2017;10:503–6.
17. Elsaie ML. Hormonal treatment of acne vulgaris: an update. Clin Cosmet Investig Dermatol. 2016;9:241–8.
18. Sardana K, Sharma RC, Sarkar R. Seasonal variation in acne vulgaris – myth or reality. J Dermatol. 2002;29(8):484–8.
19. Kathait R, Tripathi SK, Sharma SK, Shukla S. Acne: a modern skin ailment with traditional treatment. World J Pharm Pharm Sci. 2018;7(7):404–18.
20. Narasanagi S, Kuppur MSM, Shreevathsa M, Channarayapatna SKR, Kukkundur KR, Geetha N. In vitro study on anti-oxidant and anti-inflammatory properties of Varnya Mahakashaya Dashemani (aqueous extract): a polyherbal formulation. Ayu. 2018;39(2):81–6.
21. Narasanagi S, Sujnana VS, Shreevathsa M. Efficacy of Varnya Mahakashayaa Ghanavati and Churna in topical steroid-dependent face- acne rosacea- a case report. Int J Ayurvedic Herb Med. 2016;6(4):2321–5.
22. Meena V, Bhushan S, Chaudhary AK. Mugdha Rasa an ayurvedic proprietary medicine to treat acne vulgaris. Int J Green Pharm. 2017;11(4):248–52.
23. Jain A, Basal E. Inhibition of Propionibacterium acnes-induced mediators of inflammation by Indian herbs. Phytomedicine. 2003;10(1):34–8.
24. Akamatsu H, Horio T. The possible role of reactive oxygen species generated by neutrophils in mediating acne inflammation. Dermatology. 1998;196(1):82–5.
25. Chandra SD, Devendra C, Kumar SH, Meena MS. A scientific study on Rakta Dhatu and its related disorder and effect of Varnya Mahakashaya Ghanvati and Chandra Prabha Lepa in the management of Yuvan Pidika (acne vulgaris). Int J Ayurveda Pharma Res. 2014;2(2):33–9.
26. Gopal MG, Farahana B, Kulkarni KS. Effectiveness of herbal medications in the treatment of acne vulgaris – a pilot study. Indian Pract. 2001;54(10):723.
27. Paranjpe P, Kulkarni PH. Comparative efficacy of four Ayurvedic formulations in the treatment of acne vulgaris: a double-blind randomised placebo-controlled clinical evaluation. J Ethnopharmacol. 1995;49(3):127–32.

28. Thappa DM, Dogra J. Nodulocystic acne: oral gugulipid versus tetracycline. J Dermatol. 1994;21(10):729–31.
29. Dogra J, Aneja N, Saxena VN. Oral gugulipid in acne vulgaris management. Indian J Dermatol Venereol Leprol. 1990;56:381–3.
30. Agarwal RC, Singh SP, Saran RK, et al. Clinical trial of gugulipid – a new hypolipidemic agent of plant origin in primary hyperlipidemia. Indian J Med Res. 1986;84:626–34.
31. Ottaviani M, Camera E, Picardo M. Lipid mediators in acne. Mediat Inflamm. 2010;2010:858176.
32. Goyal C, Ahuja M, Sharma SK. Preparation and evaluation of anti-inflammatory activity of gugulipid-loaded proniosomal gel. Acta Pol Pharm. 2011;68(1):147–50.
33. Singh K, Chander R, Kapoor NK. Guggulsterone, a potent hypolipidaemic, prevents oxidation of low density lipoprotein. Phytother Res. 1997;11(4):291–4.
34. Sawarkar HA, Khadabadi SS, Mankar DM, Farooqui IA, Jagtap NS. Development and biological evaluation of herbal anti-acne gel. Int J Pharmtech Res. 2010;2(3):2028–31.
35. Nipanikar SU, Nagore D, Chitlange SS, Buzruk D. Evaluation of anti-inflammatory and antimicrobial activity of AHPL/AYTOP/0213 cream. Ayu. 2017;38(1–2):82–7.
36. Vijayalakshmi A, Tripura A, Ravichandiran V. Development and evaluation of anti-acne products from Terminalia arjuna bark. Int J Chemtech Res. 2003;3(1):320–7.
37. Yarnell E, Abascal K. Herbal medicine for acne vulgaris. Altern Complement Ther. 2006;12(6):303–9.
38. McMullen MK, Whitehouse JM, Towell A. Bitters: time for a new paradigm. Evid Based Complement Alternat Med. 2015;2015:670504.
39. Stokes JH, Pillsbury DM. The effect on the skin of emotional and nervous states: iii. theoretical and practical consideration of a gastro-intestinal mechanism. JAMA Dermatol. 1930;22(6):962–3.
40. Ryle JA, Barber HW. Gastric analysis in acne rosacea. Lancet. 1920;196(5076):1195–6.
41. Lombardo L, Foti M, Ruggia O, Chiecchio A. Increased incidence of small intestinal bacterial overgrowth during proton pump inhibitor therapy. Clin Gastroenterol Hepatol. 2010;8(6):504–8.
42. Clark AK, Haas KN, Sivamani RK. Edible plants and their influence on the gut microbiome and acne. Int J Mol Sci. 2017;18(5):1070.

43. Weiss E, Katta R. Diet and rosacea: the role of dietary change in the management of rosacea. Dermatol Pract Concept. 2017;7(4):31–7.
44. Ivanovska N, Philipov S. Study on the anti-inflammatory action of Berberis vulgaris root extract, alkaloid fractions and pure alkaloids. Int J Immunopharmacol. 1996;18(10):553–61.
45. Slobodnikova L, Kost'alova D, Labudova D, Kotulova D, Kettmann V. Antimicrobial activity of Mahonia aquifolium crude extract and its major isolated alkaloids. Phytother Res. 2004;18(8):674–6.
46. Seki T, Morohashi M. Effect of some alkaloids, flavonoids and triterpenoids, contents of Japanese-Chinese traditional herbal medicines, on the lipogenesis of sebaceous glands. Skin Pharmacol. 1993;6(1):56–60.
47. Clemente JC, Manasson J, Scher JU. The role of the gut microbiome in systemic inflammatory disease. BMJ. 2018;360:j5145.
48. Salem I, Ramser A, Isham N, Ghannoum MA. The gut microbiome as a major regulator of the gut-skin axis. Front Microbiol. 2018;9:1459.
49. Hacini-Rachinel F, Gheit H, Le Luduec JB, Dif F, Nancey S, Kaiserlian D. Oral probiotic control skin inflammation by acting on both effector and regulatory T cells. PLoS One. 2009;4(3):e4903.
50. Muizzuddin N, Maher W, Sullivan M, Schnittger S, Mammone T. Physiological effect of a probiotic on skin. J Cosmet Sci. 2012;63(6):385–95.
51. Kang BS, Seo JG, Lee GS, et al. Antimicrobial activity of enterocins from Enterococcus faecalis SL-5 against Propionibacterium acnes, the causative agent in acne vulgaris, and its therapeutic effect. J Microbiol. 2009;47(1):101–9.
52. Chedid V, Dhalla S, Clarke JO, Roland BC, Dunbar KB, Koh J, et al. Herbal therapy is equivalent to rifaximin for the treatment of small intestinal bacterial overgrowth. Glob Adv Health Med. 2014;3(3):16–24.
53. Lyu M, Wang YF, Fan GW, Wang XY, Xu SY, Zhu Y. Balancing herbal medicine and functional food for prevention and treatment of cardiometabolic diseases through modulating gut microbiota. Front Microbiol. 2017;8:2146.
54. Sanford JA, O'Neill AM, Zouboulis CC, Gallo RL. Short-chain fatty acids from cutibacterium acnes activate both a canonical and epigenetic inflammatory response in human sebocytes. J Immunol. 2019;202(6):1767–76.

55. Jung JY, Yoon MY, Min SU, Hong JS, Choi YS, Suh DH. The influence of dietary patterns on acne vulgaris in Koreans. Eur J Dermatol. 2010;20(6):768–72.
56. Cordain L, Lindeberg S, Hurtado M, Hill K, Eaton SB, Brand-Miller J. Acne vulgaris: a disease of Western civilization. Arch Dermatol. 2002;138(12):1584–90.
57. Smith RN, Mann NJ, Braue A, Makelainen H, Varigos GA. The effect of a high-protein, low glycemic-load diet versus a conventional, high glycemic-load diet on biochemical parameters associated with acne vulgaris: a randomized, investigator-masked, controlled trial. J Am Acad Dermatol. 2007;57(2):247–56.
58. Emiroglu N, Cengiz FP, Kemeriz F. Insulin resistance in severe acne vulgaris. Postepy Dermatol Alergol. 2015;32(4):281–5.
59. Cordain L. Implications for the role of diet in acne. Semin Cutan Med Surg. 2005;24(2):84–91.
60. Del Prete M, Mauriello MC, Faggiano A, Di Somma C, Monfrecola G, Fabbrocini G, et al. Insulin resistance and acne: a new risk factor for men? Endocrine. 2012;42(3):555–60.
61. Pedersen HK, Gudmundsdottir V, Nielsen HB, Hyotylainen T, Nielsen T, Jensen BA, et al. Human gut microbes impact host serum metabolome and insulin sensitivity. Nature. 2016;535(7612):376–81.
62. Jiminez JA, Uwiera TC, Abbott DW, Uwiera RRE, Inglis GD. Impacts of resistant starch and wheat bran consumption on enteric inflammation in relation to colonic bacterial community structures and short-chain fatty acid concentrations in mice. Gut Pathog. 2016;8:67.
63. Cani PD, Possemiers S, Van de Wiele T, et al. Changes in gut microbiota control inflammation in obese mice through a mechanism involving GLP-2-driven improvement of gut permeability. Gut. 2009;58(8):1091–103.
64. Kim YA, Keogh JB, Clifton PM. Probiotics, prebiotics, synbiotics and insulin sensitivity. Nutr Res Rev. 2018;31(1):35–51.
65. Yang J, Yin J, Gao H, Xu L, Wang Y, Xu L, et al. Berberine improves insulin sensitivity by inhibiting fat store and adjusting adipokines profile in human preadipocytes and metabolic syndrome patients. Evid Based Complement Alternat Med. 2012;2012:363845.
66. Bellamkonda R, Karuna R, Sasi Bhusana Rao B, Haritha K, Manjunatha B, Silpa S, et al. Beneficiary effect of Commiphora mukul ethanolic extract against high fructose diet induced

abnormalities in carbohydrate and lipid metabolism in wistar rats. J Tradit Complement Med. 2017;8(1):203–11.
67. Daglia M. Polyphenols as antimicrobial agents. Curr Opin Biotechnol. 2012;23(2):174–81.
68. Cowan MM. Plant products as antimicrobial agents. Clin Microbiol Rev. 1999;12(4):564–82.
69. Hutter JA, Salman M, Stavinoha WB, et al. Antiinflammatory C-glucosyl chromone from Aloe barbadensis. J Nat Prod. 1996;59(5):541–3.
70. Robson MC, Heggers JP, Hagstrom WJ. Myth, magic, witchcraft, or fact? Aloe vera revisited. J Burn Care Res. 1982;3(3):157–63.
71. Efetobor A, Odiyi BO, Falarunu LR, Abiya NU. Antimicrobial activity of three medicinal plants against acne-inducing bacteria Propionibacterium acnes. Braz J Biol Sci. 2018;5(10):277–88.
72. Kumar GS, Jayaveera KN, Kumar CK, Sanjay UP, Swamy BM, Kumar DV. Antimicrobial effects of Indian medicinal plants against acne-inducing bacteria. Trop J Pharm Res. 2007;6(2):717–23.
73. Mun SH, Joung DK, Kim YS, Kang OH, Kim SB, Seo YS, et al. Synergistic antibacterial effect of curcumin against methicillin-resistant Staphylococcus aureus. Phytomedicine. 2013;20(8–9):714–8.
74. Liu CH, Huang HY. In vitro anti-propionibacterium activity by curcumin containing vesicle system. Chem Pharm Bull (Tokyo). 2013;61(4):419–25.
75. Hegge AB, Bruzell E, Kristensen S, Tonnesen HH. Photoinactivation of Staphylococcus epidermidis biofilms and suspensions by the hydrophobic photosensitizer curcumin – effect of selected nanocarrier: studies on curcumin and curcuminoides XLVII. Eur J Pharm Sci. 2012;47(1):65–74.
76. Prasad SB, Bist M, Yashwant. In vitro anti acne activity of methanolic extract of dried fruit of Embelia ribes. Int J Pharm Qual Assur. 2018;9(1):90–4.
77. Kumar V, Bist M. Overview on anti-acne activity of methanol extract of dried fruits of Embelia ribes. Int J Sci. 2018;5(4):44–6.
78. Kumaran A, Karunakaran RJ. Nitric oxide radical scavenging active components from Phyllanthus emblica L. Plant Foods Hum Nutr. 2006;61(1):1–5.
79. Ahmad I, Beg AZ. Antimicrobial and phytochemical studies on 45 Indian medicinal plants against multi-drug resistant human pathogens. J Ethnopharmacol. 2001;74(2):113–23.

80. Kubo I, Muroi H, Kubo A. Naturally occurring antiacne agents. J Nat Prod. 1994;57(1):9–17.
81. Kumar GS, Jayaveera KN, Ashok CK. Evaluation of antioxidant and antiacne properties of terpenoidal fraction of Hemidesmus indicus (Indian sarsaparilla). Internet J Aesthet Antiag Med. 2008;1(1):1–7.
82. Chakraborty A, Brantner AH. Antibacterial steroid alkaloids from the stem bark of Holarrhena pubescens. J Ethnopharmacol. 1999;68(1–3):339–44.
83. Nam C, Kim S, Sim Y, Chang I. Anti-acne effects of oriental herb extracts: a novel screening method to select anti-acne agents. Skin Pharmacol Appl Ski Physiol. 2003;16(2):84–90.
84. Mishra A, Kumar S, Bhargava A, Sharma B, Pandey AK. Studies on in vitro antioxidant and antistaphylococcal activities of some important medicinal plants. Cell Mol Biol. 2011;57(1):16–25.
85. Patil V, Bandivadekar A, Debjani D. Inhibition of Propionibacterium acnes lipase by extracts of Indian medicinal plants. Int J Cosmet Sci. 2012;34(3):234–9.
86. Kapil A, Sharma S. Immunopotentiating compounds from Tinospora cordifolia. J Ethnopharmacol. 1997;58(2):89–95.
87. Albuquerque RG, Rocha MA, Bagatin E, Tufik S, Andersen ML. Could adult female acne be associated with modern life? Arch Dermatol Res. 2014;306(8):683–8.
88. Karl JP, Hatch AM, Arcidiacono SM, et al. Effects of psychological, environmental and physical stressors on the gut microbiota. Front Microbiol. 2018;9:2013.
89. Hassanzadeh P, Bahmani M, Mehrabani D. Bacterial resistance to antibiotics in acne vulgaris: an in vitro study. Indian J Dermatol. 2008;53(3):122–4.
90. Nakase K, Nakaminami H, Takenaka Y, Hayashi N, Kawashima M, Noguchi N. Relationship between the severity of acne vulgaris and antimicrobial resistance of bacteria isolated from acne lesions in a hospital in Japan. J Med Microbiol. 2014;63(Pt 5):721–8.
91. Meena V, Shakti Bhushan B, Chaudhary AK. Standardization of Mugdha lepa: an Ayurvedic proprietay herbo-mineral face pack for acne vulgaris. World J Pharm Res. 2017;6(16):530–9.

Chapter 11
Traditional Chinese Medicine Approaches

Valeria De Bedout and Anna J. Nichols

Introduction

Interest in complementary and alternative medicine (CAM) has significantly increased in Western countries. A 2002 report from data collected by the Centers for Disease Control and Prevention (CDC) estimated that 36% of adults in the United States used some form of CAM therapy that year [1]. CAM are a group of therapies that are used in addition to, or as an alternative to, conventional treatment. Many of those therapies lack evidence-based data to support their use [2, 3]. Traditional Chinese medicine (TCM) originated in China more than 2000 years ago, and it is one of the most common alternative therapies currently used [1, 4]. TCM is composed of a mixture of cultural philosophies, principles, and practices that include herbs,

V. De Bedout (✉)
Dr. Phillip Frost Department of Dermatology and Cutaneous Surgery, University of Miami Miller School of Medicine, Miami, FL, USA

A. J. Nichols
Clinical Trials Unit, High Risk Skin Cancer Clinic, Dr. Phillip Frost Department of Dermatology and Cutaneous Surgery, University of Miami Miller School of Medicine, Sylvester Comprehensive Cancer Center, Miami, FL, USA

R. N. Rupani, P. A. Lio (eds.), *Integrative Dermatology*,
https://doi.org/10.1007/978-3-030-58954-7_11

acupuncture, moxibustion, massage, cupping, and dietary modification [3, 5]. Patients with acne and rosacea may try CAM/TCM to reduce their personal healthcare costs, to avoid medication-associated side effects, or because they desire a more "natural" solution [6]. Acne is a chronic skin condition characterized by comedones, inflammatory papules, nodules, pustules, cysts, and scarring, mainly on the face, chest, and back [3, 4]. The cause is multifactorial, with contributions from bacterial colonization, increased sebum production, altered keratinization, hormonal imbalance, and inflammation [3, 5, 7]. Rosacea is a chronic inflammatory skin condition characterized by capillary dilation, diffuse erythema, papules, and pustules, located mainly on the cheeks and nose [8]. In this chapter, we will summarize the evidence for different forms of TCM that have been used for acne and rosacea.

Acne

Fen ci refers to the name given in Chinese to acne vulgaris, and it means *white thorns*, referring to the pustules seen in acne vulgaris [9]. TCM postulates that the cause of acne is excessive heat in the lungs or stomach, and increased moisture and blood stasis, leading to a buildup of toxins and inactivity of *qi* (vital energy) [3, 9, 10]. Therapies such as herbal medicines, acupuncture, and cupping, among others are thought to be helpful to regulate the flow of *qi*, eliminate moisture and toxins, and enhance immunologic function to induce remission in acne [3, 5, 9, 11]. Additionally, it has been thought that acupuncture may play a role in endocrine function by regulating androgen levels and thus diminishing sebum production [3]. In a 2011 study in Taiwan, 91,129 patients chose to use TCM to treat acne, and 99% of these patients used this modality as their primary therapy [5].

Herbal Remedies

Callicarpa

Callicarpa, also known as beautyberry and Zizhu, belongs to the Verbenaceae family and is known for its anti-inflammatory, hemostatic, neuroprotective, antioxidant, analgesic, and antimicrobial effects [12]. Forty-eight different species have been identified, and these are typically found in the south of China [12]. Each species of *Callicarpa* is used according to its therapeutic effects, which vary depending on its slight differences in taste and metabolites [12]. In dermatology, *Callicarpa* has been historically used for a wide variety of conditions, such as measles, furuncles and carbuncles, bruises, pruritus, desquamation, scabies, ulcers, eczema, psoriasis, and acne [12]. The anti-inflammatory, immunologic, and analgesic activities of *Callicarpa* have been studied and are attributed mainly to inhibition of cyclooxygenase-2 (COX-2), interleukin-1β (IL-1β), intercellular cell adhesion molecule-1 (ICAM-1), and vascular cell adhesion protein-1 (VCAM-1) [12]. Antioxidant activities are attributed to one of its metabolites—flavonoids—but also to its IC50 (concentration required to inhibit 50% of radical) values of hydrogen peroxide (H202) [12]. Antimicrobial effects are observed against *Staphylococcus aureus*, *Salmonella typhi*, and *Streptococcus pneumoniae* secondary to the inhibitory properties of its ethanol component [12].

In acne vulgaris, the safety profile of *Callicarpa* has been studied in 126 patients. Sixty-four patients were treated with a combination of the herbal remedy in an oral formulation plus adapalene gel (concentration was not disclosed), and 62 patients were treated only with adapalene. In terms of total lesion count, the group receiving both treatments showed better outcomes (85.94% total efficacy) compared to the control group (71.49% total efficacy), as well as fewer adverse events (10.9% vs 35.4%) [12]. In this study, oral *Callicarpa* extract was well tolerated, and side effects were mostly limited to nausea [12].

Mahonia

Mahonia belongs to the Berberidaceae family, containing 590 different species mainly found in the Northern Hemisphere and South America [13]. In dermatology, *Mahonia* root and stem have been used for the treatment of dermatitis, burns, ulcers, and acne [13]. Antimicrobial activity against *Propionibacterium acnes* (*P. acnes*) has been documented [14]. A review described the effects of *Mahonia* in a study of 92 patients with acne treated either with oral *Mahonia* or minocycline hydrochloride (dose not disclosed). In the *Mahonia* group, 31 patients displayed resolution of their acne lesions, with a total effective rate (complete clearance of lesions) of 98.28% compared to 91.18% in the control group, which was not statistically significant [13]. This implies that, in this small study, oral *Mahonia* was as at least as effective as minocycline. Larger studies are needed to confirm these findings and further investigate the safety and efficacy of *Mahonia* species for acne.

Green Tea

Green tea and specifically its polyphenols, epigallocatechin-3-gallate (EGCG) and catechin, display anticarcinogenic, anti-inflammatory, anti-lipogenic, and antimicrobial activities [7, 15, 16]. Green tea may have utility in acne vulgaris by modulating sebum production, lipogenesis, inflammation, and growth of *P. acnes* [7]. The effects of catechin have also been studied in vitro, demonstrating a reduction of the level of *P. acnes*-enhanced toll-like receptor 2 and interleukin-8, leading to a reduction in inflammation [16].

The anti-inflammatory and anti-lipogenic properties exerted by EGCG through effects on IGF-1 have been described in animal studies [15]. A study compared the effects of EGCG with all-trans retinoic acid on the sebaceous gland size in rabbits. A reduction in sebaceous gland size was evident in both groups [15].

While there is some data to suggest efficacy of EGCG and catechin in vitro and in animal studies, human studies are limited in the English literature. In a randomized, double-blind, placebo-controlled clinical trial, 80 women between the ages of 25 and 45 years with moderate to severe acne were randomized to receive either an oral preparation of 1500 mg decaffeinated green tea extract or placebo [7]. Sixty-four women completed the study. Inflammatory and noninflammatory lesion counts were recorded at baseline and 4 weeks after beginning treatment. After 4 weeks of treatment, a significant reduction in the number of inflammatory lesions was found between groups (green tea group compared to placebo group) in the following locations: nose (1.0 ± 0.8 vs 1.5 ± 1.2, p-value 0.03), perioral area (1.7 ± 1.3 vs 2.7 ± 1.9, p-value 0.04), and chin (2.3 ± 1.8 vs 3.7 ± 3.4, p-value 0.03). There were no significant between-group differences for inflammatory lesion counts in other areas, nor were there significant between-group differences for total lesion counts [7]. No major side effects were observed over the 4 weeks of the study.

Arctium lappa

Arctium lappa, also known as burdock or lappa, belongs to the Asteraceae family [17]. Historically, *Arctium lappa* roots have been used by European herbalists to treat acne because of their antioxidant, immunomodulatory, and antimicrobial properties [17]. An observational, uncontrolled interventional study evaluated the change in acne lesion count after taking oral *Arctium lappa* 6c (potency), four pills of 40 size, four times a day for 1 week, followed by placebo for one additional week, in 32 subjects (20 men and 12 women) [17]. The 1-week treatment was not repeated, but patients were followed for 6 months. Outcome was assessed by a homeopathic doctor using the Global Acne Grading System to identify the type and number of lesions. A statistically significant improvement in total inflammatory and noninflammatory lesion count was observed, with a total lesion count at baseline of 20.3 compared to 10 at the end of the study (p-value 0.001), potentially due to the antimicrobial properties of lappa against *P. acnes* [17].

Myrica rubra

Myrica rubra, also known as bayberry, belongs to the Myricaceae family, and it is known for its antimicrobial properties against *P. acnes* [18]. Its antioxidant and anti-inflammatory effects on sebocytes stimulated by *P. acnes* have been studied in vitro, and it has been shown to be effective at suppressing *P. acnes*-induced cytokine production by regulating toll-like receptors [18]. No human studies have been reported in the English literature for *Myrica rubra* as a treatment for acne.

Combination Preparations

Oftentimes, a preparation of multiple herbs is given to patients in order to take advantage of potential synergistic effects [19, 20]. The preparations consist of a mixture of herbs such as those previously mentioned, plus *Oldenlandia diffusa*, *Angelica*, *Sophora flavescens*, and others [19, 20]. Examples of these preparations include *Zhen Ren Huo Ming Yin*, *Huang Lian Jie Du Tang*, *Tuo Li Xiao Du Yin*, *Wen Qing Yin*, *Gan Lu Yin*, *Pi Pa Qing Fei Yin*, *Fu Fang She She Cao He Ji*, *Dang Gui Ku Shen Wan*, and *Tao Hong Si Wu Tang* [9, 19]. In TCM, it is thought that when acne is caused by excessive heat in the lungs and stomach, oily skin, dry mouth, thirst, and constipation result. For these patients, a combination of herbs known as *Pi Pa Qing Fei Yin* and *Dan Di Tang* is often used [9]. Several small studies have evaluated the efficacy of such formulations for the treatment of acne vulgaris and acneiform drug reactions secondary to medications, such as epidermal growth factor receptor (EGFR) inhibitors [19, 20]. Preparations that claim to be antimicrobial include a mix of kampo extracts known as *Keigairengyoto*, *Huang Lian*

(Rhizoma coptidis), and *Gan Cao* (Radix glycyrrhizae), which have been shown to be effective against *P. acnes* and *S. epidermidis*, possibly secondary to its antioxidant actions on infiltrated neutrophils [21–23]. In a case–control study evaluating 120 men and women with acne vulgaris, the treatment group (86 subjects) received a compounded mixture of oldenlandis in a dose of 200 mg twice daily, while the control group (34 subjects) were treated with *Dang Gui Ku Shen Wan* orally at a dose of 6 grams twice daily. The treatment group had a reported cure rate (defined as disappearance of all acne lesions) of 44.19% compared to 29.41% in the control group (p-value < 0.05) [20].

The most commonly reported side effects in patients with acne treated with these herbal remedies include dizziness, nausea, abdominal pain, diarrhea, pruritus, dryness, and burning sensation [3, 5, 20].

Acupuncture

Acupuncture is one of the TCM modalities that dates back to ancient China, and consists of inserting solid thin needles in specific points in the skin, with the aim of correcting an imbalanced flow of *qi* through channels known as meridians [6, 9, 11]. The use of acupuncture in dermatology has been widely used in China, and patients with acne often pursue this treatment [24–27]. The most common acupoints for acne are *Hegu* (LI 4), *Quchi* (LI 11), *Yinlingquan* (SP 9), *Xuehai* (SP 10), *Sanyinjiao* (SP 6), *Zusanli* (ST 36), *Taichong* (LR 3), *Zhongwan* (CV 12), *Tianshu* (ST 25), *Shangxing* (GV 23), *Taiyang* (EX-HN5), and *Yangbai* (GB 14) [10]. A study compared the efficacy of acupuncture with helium–neon laser with a power density of 25 mW/cm^2 for the treatment of acne vulgaris. Sixty-eight patients (both men and women) were divided into two groups, one treated with helium–neon laser auricular irradiation (20 min per session for a total of ten sessions on predetermined auricular points with a distance of 30–50 cm from the skin) plus acupuncture (once daily for ten sessions) and the other group treated only with acupuncture (once daily for ten sessions). The acupoints used in the acupuncture sessions were LI4, LI11, GV23, EX-HN5, ST36, and GB14.The combination of laser plus acupuncture was more effective, with a cure rate defined as complete disappearance of acne lesions, of 77.8% in the treatment group compared to 46.9% in the control group [10]. A Cochrane database systematic review summarized the results of two studies that evaluated the efficacy of acupuncture in the treatment of acne and compared this approach to traditional Western medicine therapies. Neither of these individual studies is available in the English literature, but according to the systematic review, the treatment of acne vulgaris with acupuncture vs oral antibiotics or oral retinoids proved to be similar among groups, with no statistical inferiority of acupuncture compared to Western medicine [3]. Adverse effects have not been widely studied, but pruritus, erythema, contact dermatitis, and pain are the most commonly reported symptoms after acupuncture therapy [3].

Cupping

Cupping is a technique that consists of suctioning skin areas in order to mobilize blood flow and promote healing [11]. The efficacy of cupping for the treatment of acne has been studied alone and compared with retinoids, oral tetracyclines, and herbal preparations [3]. A Cochrane database systematic review described a study not available in the English literature that compared the acne remission rate of cupping with oral tetracycline in 60 subjects (men and women). The *ashi points* (defined as points that are needled based on where patients have pain or where there is obvious inflammation) in the first lateral line of the bladder channel on the back were pricked ten times with a three-edged needle to identify the ideal sites for cupping (points that bled). Cupping was then used only on those sites once a day for a total of ten treatments over 1 month. Achromycin 1 gram daily was given to the control group during the same period of time. Remission was defined as clearance of 95% or more of the lesions with only mild hyperpigmentation and scars remaining. A statistically significant improvement was observed in patients treated with cupping (RR 2.50, 95% CI 1.31–4.77, $p = 0.005$) [3]. Skin bruising and discoloration were the most commonly reported side effects [3].

Diet

Diet is an important component of TCM. Chinese medical theory states that an unhealthy diet could immediately cause imbalances and thus, when treating acne, a strict *yin* or *yang* diet is recommended, which is focused on a balanced diet [28]. *Yin* foods are generally cold, low in calories, and high in potassium, whereas *yang* foods are believed to be warm and dry. It is thought that balance or equilibrium should be maintained between *yin* and *yang* for ideal health. Cereals, legumes, vegetables, soups, and algae are in the center (equilibrium) and represent the base of a traditional Chinese diet, whereas alcohol, sugar, dairy, eggs, and meat are to be consumed sparingly or avoided completely. A cross-sectional study performed in China evaluated the acne severity and *yin* and *yang* diet scores using a quantitative method in 322 patients. Experts evaluated each subject's diet in an attempt to correlate their *yin* and *yang* diet to their signs and symptoms. *Yin* refers to pale skin and tongue color, deep pulse, and low activity or energy, whereas *yang* refers to brightly colored or red tongue and a high level of activity. After this assessment, a score was assigned to each subject on a scale of minus 10 to plus 10 (where zero represents a state of balance), and thus a *yin* or *yang* predominance was established. The authors found that in patients predominantly following a *yin* diet, a lower incidence of acne was observed. Those following a *yang* diet were found to have a higher incidence of acne [28]. Two additional randomized controlled trials assessed dietary interventions in patients with acne [29, 30]. Low-glycemic index diets were compared with high-glycemic index diets in patients with acne. Smith et al. studied 43 men with acne in a randomized controlled study where the treatment group consisted of a low-glycemic diet comprised of 25% protein and 45% low-glycemic index carbohydrates, whereas the control group consisted of a dense-glycemic diet. Acne lesion counts and acne lesion severity were assessed at 12 weeks. The total acne lesion count significantly decreased in the low-glycemic diet group compared to the high-glycemic diet group (−23.5 + −3.9 vs −12.0 + −3.5 $p = 0.03$) [30]. Similarly, Kwon et al. studied the effects of a low-glycemic load diet in 32 patients (men and women) with mild to moderate acne who were randomly assigned either to a low-glycemic load diet or a control group diet for 10 weeks [29]. Only patients in the intervention group displayed a significant improvement both in their inflammatory and noninflammatory lesions, with acne scores (performed by dermatologists using the Leeds revised acne grading system and digital photography) changing from 2.18 to 1.6 ($p = 0.02$) [29].

Rosacea

Similar to acne, Chinese medicine theorizes that rosacea is related to blood heat, blood stasis, and accumulation of heat in the lungs and stomach. Hence, the basic treatment principle is to dissipate heat in those areas, remove toxic substances, and activate blood circulation [8]. Herbal remedies and acupuncture are the two most commonly used TCM modalities for rosacea.

Herbal Remedies

Individual herbs and combinations of different preparations have been reported to be effective for the treatment of rosacea. A preparation known as CBX (consisting of loquat leaf, mulberry bark, *Scutellaria* root, *Imperata* rhizome, red peony root, safflower, red sage, chuanxiong, Dahurian angelica, motherwort, and Chinese trumpet creeper flower) is believed to be effective for dissipating heat and, thus, treating rosacea [8]. Specifically, safflower, red sage root, and chuanxiong are believed to activate blood circulation and thus remove toxins [8]. One case–control study evaluated the effect of CBX preparation in 68 women with rosacea. All patients were treated with spironolactone 60 mg/day plus minocycline 100 mg/day; 48 of those patients additionally received CBX orally twice daily for 8 weeks. The patients in the CBX group had a reported cure rate of 87.5%, when compared to a cure rate of 45% in the control group with a p-value < 0.01 [8]. Cure rate was defined in this study as remission of 90% or more of lesions including erythema, papules, pustules, and capillary dilation.

Acupuncture

Acupuncture may be a valuable tool for the treatment of rosacea; however, there is a paucity of data to support this approach in the English literature [11, 31]. One reported case describes a patient treated with three acupuncture sessions over 1 week, with needles inserted into the acupoints of Yintang (EX-HN3), bilateral Taiyang (EX-HN5), bilateral Yingxiang (LI20), and Chengjiang (CV 24). She was then followed for 6 months and demonstrated a substantial and sustained improvement in her rosacea, without recurrence [31].

Conclusion

A large proportion of patients are interested in complementary and alternative medicine in general, and traditional Chinese medicine in particular, thus healthcare practitioners should be aware of TCM theory, therapeutic modalities, potential mechanisms of action, and possible side effects. There is still a lack of evidence-based research on this topic.

Well-designed, larger randomized controlled studies with longer follow-up are needed in order to evaluate their safety and efficacy. Head-to-head studies comparing these modalities to the available therapies used in Western medicine would be most useful. The available literature demonstrates the potential relevance of TCM for the treatment of dermatological conditions, including acne and rosacea, and how TCM could be used as a complement to Western medicine.

References

1. Barnes PM, Powell-Griner E, McFann K, Nahin RL. Complementary and alternative medicine use among adults: United States, 2002. Adv Data. 2004;27(343):1–19.
2. Verhoef MJ, Hilsden RJ, O'Beirne M. Complementary therapies and cancer care: an overview. Patient Educ Couns. 1999;38(2):93–100.
3. Cao H, Yang G, Wang Y, Liu JP, Smith CA, Luo H, et al. Complementary therapies for acne vulgaris. Cochrane Database Syst Rev. 2015;1:CD009436.
4. Chen FP, Chen TJ, Kung YY, Chen YC, Chou LF, Chen FJ, et al. Use frequency of traditional Chinese medicine in Taiwan. BMC Health Serv Res. 2007;7:26.
5. Chen HY, Lin YH, Chen YC. Identifying Chinese herbal medicine network for treating acne: implications from a nationwide database. J Ethnopharmacol. 2016;179:1–8.
6. Iliev E. Acupuncture in dermatology. Clin Dermatol. 1998;16(6):659–88.
7. Lu PH, Hsu CH. Does supplementation with green tea extract improve acne in post-adolescent women? A randomized, double-blind, and placebo-controlled clinical trial. Complement Ther Med. 2016;25:159–63.
8. Yu TG, Zheng YZ, Zhu JT, Guo W. Effect of treatment of rosacea in females by Chibixiao recipe in combination with minocycline and spironolactone. Chin J Integr Med. 2006;12(4):277–80.
9. Baroni A, Ruocco E, Russo T, Piccolo V, Geng L, Zhou H, et al. The use of traditional Chinese medicine in some dermatologic diseases: part I--acne, psoriasis, and atopic dermatitis. Skinmed. 2015;13(1):32–8; quiz 9.

10. Lihong S. He-Ne laser auricular irradiation plus body acupuncture for treatment of acne vulgaris in 36 cases. J Tradit Chin Med. 2006;26(3):193–4.
11. Tan EK, Millington GW, Levell NJ. Acupuncture in dermatology: an historical perspective. Int J Dermatol. 2009;48(6):648–52.
12. Tu Y, Sun L, Guo M, Chen W. The medicinal uses of Callicarpa L. in traditional Chinese medicine: an ethnopharmacological, phytochemical and pharmacological review. J Ethnopharmacol. 2013;146(2):465–81.
13. He JM, Mu Q. The medicinal uses of the genus Mahonia in traditional Chinese medicine: an ethnopharmacological, phytochemical and pharmacological review. J Ethnopharmacol. 2015;175:668–83.
14. Slobodnikova L, Kost'alova D, Labudova D, Kotulova D, Kettmann V. Antimicrobial activity of Mahonia aquifolium crude extract and its major isolated alkaloids. Phytother Res. 2004;18(8):674–6.
15. Im M, Kim SY, Sohn KC, Choi DK, Lee Y, Seo YJ, et al. Epigallocatechin-3-gallate suppresses IGF-I-induced lipogenesis and cytokine expression in SZ95 sebocytes. J Invest Dermatol. 2012;132(12):2700–8.
16. Jung MK, Ha S, Son JA, Song JH, Houh Y, Cho E, et al. Polyphenon-60 displays a therapeutic effect on acne by suppression of TLR2 and IL-8 expression via down-regulating the ERK1/2 pathway. Arch Dermatol Res. 2012;304(8):655–63.
17. Miglani A, Manchanda RK. Observational study of Arctium lappa in the treatment of acne vulgaris. Homeopathy. 2014;103(3):203–7.
18. Chen KC, Yang CH, Li TT, Zouboulis CC, Huang YC. Suppression of Propionibacterium acnes-stimulated proinflammatory cytokines by Chinese bayberry extracts and its active constituent myricetin in human sebocytes in vitro. Phytother Res. 2019;33(4):1104–13.
19. Hung YC, Chin CY, Lee YC, Chen YH, Tsai MY. Clinical experience of Chinese herbal medicine ameliorates dermatologic events from epidermal growth factor receptor inhibitors for lung cancer: a case series. Explore (NY). 2019;15(5):363–70.
20. Liu W, Shen D, Song P, Xu X. Clinical observation in 86 cases of acne vulgaris treated with compound Oldenlandis mixture. J Tradit Chin Med. 2003;23(4):255–6.
21. Higaki S, Morimatsu S, Morohashi M, Yamagishi T, Hasegawa Y. Susceptibility of Propionibacterium acnes, Staphylococcus

aureus and Staphylococcus epidermidis to 10 Kampo formulations. J Int Med Res. 1997;25(6):318–24.
22. Kim KS, Kim YB. Interaction and efficacy of Keigai-rengyo-to extract and acupuncture in male patients with acne vulgaris: a study protocol for a randomized controlled pilot trial. Trials. 2011;12:82.
23. Nam C, Kim S, Sim Y, Chang I. Anti-acne effects of oriental herb extracts: a novel screening method to select anti-acne agents. Skin Pharmacol Appl Ski Physiol. 2003;16(2):84–90.
24. Liu J. Treatment of adolescent acne with acupuncture. J Tradit Chin Med. 1993;13(3):187–8.
25. Chen D, Jiang N, Cong X. 47 cases of acne treated by prick-bloodletting plus cupping. J Tradit Chin Med. 1993;13(3):185–6.
26. Xu Y. Treatment of facial skin diseases with acupuncture--a report of 129 cases. J Tradit Chin Med. 1990;10(1):22–5.
27. Ding LN. 50 cases of acne treated by puncturing acupoint dazhui in combination with cupping. J Tradit Chin Med. 1985;5(2):128.
28. Law MP, Chuh AA, Molinari N, Lee A. An investigation of the association between diet and occurrence of acne: a rational approach from a traditional Chinese medicine perspective. Clin Exp Dermatol. 2010;35(1):31–5.
29. Kwon HH, Yoon JY, Hong JS, Jung JY, Park MS, Suh DH. Clinical and histological effect of a low glycaemic load diet in treatment of acne vulgaris in Korean patients: a randomized, controlled trial. Acta Derm Venereol. 2012;92(3):241–6.
30. Smith RN, Mann NJ, Braue A, Makelainen H, Varigos GA. A low-glycemic-load diet improves symptoms in acne vulgaris patients: a randomized controlled trial. Am J Clin Nutr. 2007;86(1):107–15.
31. Gao Y, Lin W, Zhou S, Shi G, He J, Chen Y. Treatment of Rosacea using acupuncture for improving the local skin microcirculation: a case report. Medicine (Baltimore). 2018;97(34):e11931.

Chapter 12
Homeopathy in the Therapy of Acne and Rosacea

Lawrence Chukwudi Nwabudike

Introduction

Homeopathy is a holistic system of integrative medicine based on the "law of similars." It was founded by the German physician Samuel Christian Hahnemann (10 April 1755–2 July 1843) and one of his first essays on the subject was published in 1796 [1]. However, his work *Organon der Heilkunst* (*Organon of Medicine*) details many of the principles of the therapeutic system named "homeopathy" by him [2]. This was first published in 1810 [1] and revised several times [2]. Homeopathy is based on the principle that serial dilution and succussion (vigorous shaking with banging on a hard surface) "potentizes" (increases the strength) the solution, as well as imprints the "essence" of the medicine on the "memory" of water. Many remain skeptical, as the dilutions are often so high that, based on the Avogadro number, not a single molecule of the original substance should exist in a homeopathic solution. Yet this theory of imprinting of water appears to have found some support in research showing the existence of nanomolecules in homeopathic solutions [3, 4].

L. C. Nwabudike (✉)
Department of Outpatient Dermatology, N. Paulescu National Institute of Diabetes, Bucharest, Romania

R. N. Rupani, P. A. Lio (eds.), *Integrative Dermatology*,
https://doi.org/10.1007/978-3-030-58954-7_12

These nanomolecules appear to be formed from the water itself and may even mimic the electromagnetic signature of the original substance.

The principle of similars espoused by Hahnemann means that a substance that, at one concentration, may produce certain symptoms of disease in a healthy individual may also treat those symptoms in a sick one [2]. Thus, homeopaths try to match disease presentations to the symptoms of various homeopathic medicines. This matching medicine is known as the similimum.

Principles of Treatment

Homeopathy seeks to treat the patient as an individual entity, rather than to treat the physical disease alone. However, disease-specific homeopathic treatments are also widely used. Homeopathic medications—homeopaths also refer to them as "remedies"—are used in different dilutions. As a general principle, the lower dilutions are used more for physical ailments and the higher dilutions used for a deeper effect, which would have an effect on both the physical body and the psyche. Dilutions generally begin from a mother tincture and dilutions are made serially; thus, a 1C potency is a 1:100 dilution; the 2C potency is made with a 1 part 1C solution diluted in 99 parts alcohol and is a 1:10,000 dilution, etc.; a 6C solution = 1:1000,000,000,000; a 13C dilution, according to the Avogadro number, no longer has any molecules of the original solution. Each dilution is followed by vigorous shaking, known as a succussion, which is thought to "potentize" the solution. As a result of these extremely high dilutions, in which there are no molecules of the original substance, homeopathic medicines are thought to lack the potential for allergic or teratogenic effects.

In homeopathy, acne and rosacea are considered chronic diseases, i.e., diseases that have a deep underlying cause, based on the individual constitution. The homeopathic consultation in such cases aims to uncover this underlying individual picture and match it to the symptom picture of a particular medicine. Typical questions in such a consultation would cover the psychological profile of the patient—"mental" symptoms as homeopaths call them—and the physical symptoms. Questions that cover the psychological profile might include fears, e.g., of heights, narrow places, unknown, failure, etc., and fastidiousness/non-fastidiousness and reaction when angry/upset, when consoled, and when contradicted, among others. The order in which the disease appeared, forehead first, then cheeks, etc.; lateralization (simply meaning which side is predominantly worse "left/right"); aggravating/ameliorating factors—emotions, ambient temperature, pressure, etc. and food likes/aversions—thirst/lack of thirst; sleep patterns; and menstruation patterns, among others are also included in the physical symptoms.

The profiles of homeopathic medications can be found in the homeopathic *materia medicae*, while symptoms and symptom combinations are found in what homeopaths refer to as homeopathic repertories. Combinations of symptoms help homeopaths arrive at a matching therapy. In more recent times, sophisticated computer programs have been developed to help rapidly combine these symptoms so as to arrive more quickly at potential therapeutic approaches.

Efforts have been made to standardize and improve the quality of homeopathic case reporting. Some of this has crystalized in the HOM-CASE guidelines [5], developed along the lines of the CARE guidelines for case reporting. In order to aid more critical analysis of cases and to improve their quality, the modified Naranjo criteria have been proposed [5], after the original Naranjo criteria, in order to define the probability of causality between the administered homeopathic medicine and the changes observed in the patient. Table 12.1 gives the modified Naranjo criteria proposed for case descriptions [5], while Tables 12.2 and 12.3 give the scores based on the modified Naranjo criteria.

Homeopathy is the second most common form of CAM/integrative medicine therapy used by dermatology outpatients, up to 37.9% of individuals [6]. Acne and rosacea are

TABLE 12.1 Modified Naranjo criteria [5] with permission

Criterion number	Criterion definition	Yes	No	Not sure or not applicable (N/A)
1	Was there an improvement in the main symptom or condition for which the homeopathic medicine was prescribed?	+2	−1	0
2	Did the clinical improvement occur within a plausible time frame relative to the drug intake?	+1	−2	0
3	Was there an initial aggravation of symptoms?	+1	0	0
4	Did the effect encompass more than the main symptom or condition, i.e., were other symptoms ultimately improved or changed?	+1	0	0
5	Did overall well-being improve?	+1	0	0
6a	Direction of cure: did some symptoms improve in the opposite order of the development of symptoms of the disease?	+1	0	0
6b	Direction of cure: did *at least two* of the following aspects apply to the order of improvement of symptoms: • from organs of more importance to those of less importance • from deeper to more superficial aspects of the individual • and from the top downward?	+1	0	0

TABLE 12.1 (continued)

Criterion number	Criterion definition	Yes	No	Not sure or not applicable (N/A)
7	Did "old symptoms" (defined as nonseasonal and noncyclical symptoms that were previously thought to have resolved) reappear temporarily during the course of improvement?	+1	0	0
8	Are there any alternative causes (other than the medicine) that, with a high probability, could have caused the improvement (consider known course of disease, other forms of treatment and other clinically relevant interventions)?	−3	+1	0
9	Was the health improvement confirmed by any objective evidence (e.g., lab test, clinical observation, etc.)?	+2	0	0
10	Did repeat dosing, if conducted, create similar clinical improvement?	+1	0	0

Highest score is 13, least is 3

among the most common skin disorders treated with CAM (24% and 6.9%, respectively) [6]. Homeopathy use has been estimated at 2.1% of the adult US population and may be increasing [7].

Evidence suggests that more than 80% of physicians wish to have knowledge that would allow them to have meaningful discussions with their patients regarding CAM [8]. This work hopes to help fill this knowledge gap.

Acne and Homeopathy

Acne is a chronic skin disorder with significant potential for reduction in patients' quality of life. A variety of conventional therapies exist and are discussed in a therapeutic guideline for acne [9]. Some of those discussed and suggested as potentially useful treatments in this guideline include tea tree oil, biofeedback, and herbs. The authors of this guideline conclude that there is some evidence of efficacy [9].

The efficacy of *Zingiber officinale* (ginger) in the therapy of acne was assessed in a prospective, non-randomized, open-labeled study [10]. Study population was 31 patients (with 32 patients enrolled and 1 dropout) using homeopathic potencies of 6C to 1 M. The potencies were increased based on response, i.e., if 6C gave no response or no longer produced effect, then 30C, 200C, and 1 M were administered. Primary outcomes were percentage of change of lesion count and Global Acne Grading System (GAGS) score at 6 months. Acne-specific quality-of-life (Acne-QoL) scores as well as changes in identified homeopathic symptoms and signs were secondary endpoints. Participants showed improvement in inflammatory lesion counts (mean 107 to 46), GAGS (mean 19 to 10) scores, and Acne-QoL scores (60.4 to 88.2), with no deterioration in any of the enrolled patients. The authors concluded that homeopathic *Zingiber officinale* was efficacious in the treatment of acne, but larger studies with placebo control would be required to confirm their results.

Zingiber officinale has been studied extensively and the European Medicines Agency (EMA) lists its effects as being anti-inflammatory, anti-infectious, and antineoplastic, among others [11]. With regard to homeopathy, some authors suggest the use of *Zingiber officinale* for large, erythematous acne lesions, usually worse on the left side [12].

An uncontrolled, observational, interventional study was conducted using *Arctium lappa* (greater burdock) in patients with acne [13]. Thirty-four patients were enrolled, and two patients dropped out (one due to pregnancy and the other due to antibiotic therapy for another disorder). Patients received *Arctium lappa* at potencies of 6C–1 M. Each potency was given four times a day for 7 days, and then placebo was administered for further 7 days. If no improvement was seen, the regimen was repeated, with a higher potency, but thrice daily. Treatment was for a 6-month period. The reason for the change from four times daily to three times daily use of medicine was not clear from the methodology. Endpoints were change in lesion counts, GAGS scores, and Acne-QoL scores. The results showed significant reduction in lesion counts (mean 157 to 59) and GAGS scores (mean 20.3 to 10), with improvement of Acne-QoL scores (mean 63 to 90.7). The authors concluded that *Arctium lappa* could be effective as a treatment for acne, though larger, controlled studies would be needed to confirm these results.

Arctium lappa is a plant native to the Eurasian region. It is grown widely as a garden plant and as a vegetable. It has been used in traditional Chinese medicine for purifying the blood and improving blood flow to the skin surface [14]. The European Medicines Agency (EMA) lists it as a herbal medicine useful for seborrheic (oily) skin, which may explain its value in acne [15]. A homeopathic text lists *Arctium lappa* as being useful for acne; hyperhidrosis with offensive odor, chiefly in the axillary region; as well as pustular and eczematous rashes [16].

Azadirachta indica (Indian lilac, neem) is a member of the mahogany family and is a tree native to the Indian subcontinent. It is an ancient remedy that has been used widely in Ayurveda and Chinese medicine. It has anti-inflammatory, free radical scavenging, anticancer, and antibacterial effects [17]. In homeopathy, *Azadirachta indica* has been of value for pustular eruptions, eczema, skin ulcers, amnesia, depression, and even leprosy [16].

Azadirachta indica was tested in an open-label, prospective, observational study of 31 patients [18]. *Azadirachta indica* was administered at potencies from 6C to 1 M, initially four times per day for 7 weeks, followed by placebo. The medication was repeated at the same potency if the improvement appeared to be slowed. If there was no further improvement, then 30C, 200C, and 1 M potencies were administered in the same manner, but at three times daily dosage, for 1 week, followed by placebo.

Outcomes were change in lesion count, GAGS scores, and Acne-QoL scores. Results showed decrease in average lesion count (128 to 82) and GAGS scores (23 to 20) and improved Acne-QoL scores (71.03 to 88.48) that were all significant. The authors conclude that, although their results suggested that *Azadirachta indica* showed efficacy in acne, this efficacy would need to be confirmed by more rigorous studies.

Homeopathic *Sulphur* and *Tuberculinum* were tested in a placebo-controlled, non-blinded, observational study involving patients with acne scars [19]. The patients were divided into two groups (100 treated group and 20 placebo group). Although the authors reported a 92% improvement in the treated group and 20% improvement in the placebo group, the description of the methodology does not state medication potency and mode of administration, as well as which of the two medicines was more effective. The results appear to suggest that homeopathy may be effective in the treatment of acne scars. Both homeopathic *Sulphur* and *Tuberculinum* are widely used for skin diseases in general. A significant limitation of the applicability of this study is that the potency of the medications used in this study was not specified. Studies with clearer methodology might better elucidate the role of homeopathy in the treatment of acne scars.

A retrospective study of 83 patients treated with classical (individualized) homeopathy was carried out [20]. The patients were prescribed the homeopathic medicine that most corresponded to them as individuals at 1 M and occasionally C200 potency (usually where M potency was unavailable), on a weekly basis. The patients were followed up at 6- to 8-week intervals. The patients were also followed up photographically, with corresponding consent, and divided into mild (comedones), moderate (inflammatory and noninflammatory lesions), and severe (pustules, cysts, and nodules). Results were classified as remission, failure, and lost to follow-up (LTF). The results showed a remission rate of 81.9%, 2.4% failed treatment, and 15.7% LTF. Average time to remission was 1.9 months (range 1.5–6 months), with no relapse and no side effects recorded. The most commonly prescribed medicines, based on analysis of the raw data, were *Lycopodium clavatum* (38.6%), *Palladium metallicum* (15.6%), and *Platinum metallicum* (12.0%). The author concluded that individualized homeopathic treatment could be efficacious in treating acne, but larger studies and more rigorous methodology would be required to confirm this.

A case study of individualized homeopathic medicines with acne ($n = 2$) was reported [21]. The patients were aged 14 and 16 years with severe pustular acne and received the homeopathic medicines *Palladium metallicum* C200 potency and *Natrum muriaticum* 1 M potency, given at weekly intervals. The patients showed complete remission, with improvement in acne scars.

For both studies of individualized homeopathic treatment of acne, a potential confounder would be the level of skill of the practitioner. Individualized homeopathic prescribing often requires a high degree of experience on the part of the prescriber to optimize therapy. Such studies are very difficult, if not impossible, to carry out with placebo control, making studies with a high level of evidence much more scarce.

First Case Description

A 13-year-old female patient presented with a 2-year history of facial and truncal rash. There was no significant medical history. Physical examination showed erythematous papules and pustules, as well as atrophic scars predominantly on the face and trunk (Fig. 12.1a). There was no lateralization of physical signs. The patient was thirsty, not desirous of open spaces, and was not chilly.

From the homeopathic standpoint, the patient loved company, loved admiration, and was willing to make compromises to achieve them; she was averse to consolation, lacked self-confidence, was not intolerant to contradiction, and had no fear of heights or narrow spaces.

Following a homeopathic consultation, the patient was prescribed homeopathic *Palladium metallicum* C200 potency, weekly administration. Homeopathic differential diagnoses included *Pulsatilla* and *Platinum metallicum. Pulsatilla* also lacks confidence, but desires consolation and usually leans on others for psychological support, especially when making decisions. *Pulsatilla* also desires consolation and will actively seek it. *Pulsatilla* has been described as chilly and is usually thirstless. Thus, weeping in public is an option with *Pulsatilla*, maybe with *Palladium metallicum*, never with *Platinum metallicum. Platinum metallicum*, like the other two homeopathic medicines, is a female-specific medicine. It has often been described as haughty, as the combination of its desire for admiration, without compromising herself (great pride), gives this image. *Platinum metallicum* desires company and is usually averse to solitude; dislike for/fear of narrow places, unknown, as well as failure; and can be fastidious. *Platinum metallicum* is usually not chilly and more frequently right sided in lateralization. All three medicines have a deep lack of self-confidence. It appears "convenient" for *Pulsatilla*, accepted by *Palladium metallicum* and must not show in *Platinum metallicum*. For this reason, *Platinum metallicum* is intolerant to contradiction. These two characteristics do not appear to feature prominently with *Palladium metallicum* and *Pulsatilla*.

The patient was in remission by the 6-week visit, with decreased number of lesions, reduced erythema, and marked reduction in frequency of new lesions. By 1 year after initiation of treatment (Fig. 12.1b), the patient had no more acne lesions and also showed improvement of scars. Remission continued after the cessation of homeopathic medicine, though the patient no longer came personally for therapy.

The homeopathic assessment of a patient with acne treated with homeopathy will include the assessment of the physical complaint as well as an assessment of the "mental" symptoms of the patient, i.e., the psychological characteristics that help define the patient as corresponding to one medicine or the other. It is also necessary to take into consideration how the ailment affects the patient's life. Often patients with acne present hoping for rapid responses; they

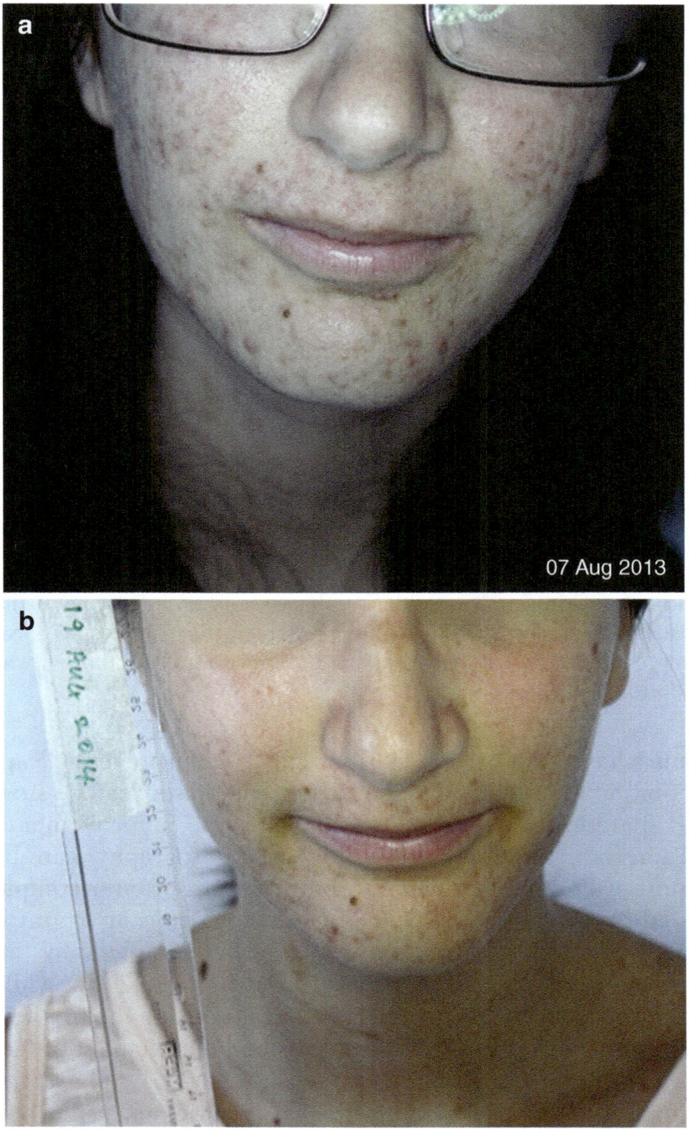

FIGURE 12.1 (**a**) Before onset of treatment, patient with facial papules, pustules, and scars. (**b**) At 1 year after onset of treatment, lesions cleared and scars improved

Table 12.2 Modified Naranjo criteria for the first case description

Criterion	Points allocated
1	+2
2	+1
3	+1
4	+1
5	+1
6a	0
6b	0
7	0
8	+1
9	+2
10	+1
Total	+8

Note: for Criterion 8, considering the severity and duration of the patient's acne, it is not "highly probable" that she would have improved without some form of therapy. Therefore, the +1 was allotted instead of –3

must have proper expectations set to help prevent disappointment. Often, the response to homeopathy can be slow, so patients may not easily notice the improvements. Therefore, baseline and follow-up photography can be quite useful. Homeopathic treatments are often accompanied by the homeopathic aggravation, which is an aggravation of the physical symptoms, accompanied by an amelioration of the psychological symptoms. Thus, while there may be an increase in acne lesions during the first few weeks of treatment, there is usually an improvement of factors such as sleep, emotional state, etc. This follows the homeopathic principle that healing goes from inside out. Homeopathic aggravations may sometimes go unnoticed by the patient. Their presence is usually a good indication that the selected medicine is the right one.

Rosacea and Homeopathy

A significant proportion of patients (6.9%) using CAM for skin conditions use it for the therapy of rosacea [6]. There is a dearth of studies related to the therapy of rosacea with homeopathy in the literature. The reasons for this, in comparison with acne, are not immediately obvious.

One case study (*n* = 3) of individualized homeopathic treatment of rosacea [22] included two females and one male, age range 32–53 years. They suffered from erythematotelangiectatic and papulopustular forms of rosacea. The homeopathic medicines used were *Causticum*, *Lachesis muta*, and *Lycopodium clavatum*, all at 1 M potency, given on a weekly basis. Time to remission was 6 weeks. The patients remained in remission after cessation of treatment.

Causticum is homeopathic potassium hydroxide. The mental picture is one of an activist, always fighting injustice. They are extremely sympathetic to the sufferings of others, so *Causticum* would lend a helping hand to the homeless or stray animals, and may sometimes even do co-workers' work for them, in order to spare them from suffering. *Causticum* can be irritable also and is very anxious about the well-being of loved ones. *Causticum* is chilly, with left lateralization, and is constipated. The constipation of *Causticum* is characterized by a lack of urge, and sometimes, in children, peculiarly, they need to stand to pass feces. Clinically, *Causticum* suffers from warts and paresis, usually mononeuropathy, thus has been useful for carpal tunnel syndrome and various palsies.

Lachesis muta is derived from the venom of the bushmaster snake with the same name, which is a part of the pit viper family. *Lachesis muta* is a very competitive individual. Jealousy is a keynote symptom and *Lachesis muta* individuals are always pushing boundaries of rules. They are averse to anything that poses limitations, unless set by them. This may explain the characteristic aversion of *Lachesis muta* individuals to narrow spaces and to wearing tight clothing (especially belts and ties). They are averse to heat and are usually lateralized to the left. As a result of their difficulty with boundaries, they can fall into alcoholism or excessive sex. Clinically, *Lachesis muta* is useful for hot flushes and hemorrhagic disorders such as nose bleeds, menorrhagia, ecchymoses/purpura and necrotic skin lesions.

Lycopodium clavatum is a plant-based medicine. A keynote of *Lycopodium clavatum* is vulnerability. It is a medicine that feels inwardly small, wishes to be big, and is afraid this vulnerability might be discovered. *Lycopodium clavatum* therefore has fear of/aversion to the unknown, public speaking, and unprepared interviews (or any situation with potential for exposing these weaknesses); intolerance of contradiction, though not necessarily wanting to lead; and aversion to solitude (though for *Lycopodium clavatum* company is more useful for its presence rather than its human value); it is a right-sided medicine, may or may not be chilly, and tends to be constipated (especially in unfamiliar places, during travels, etc.). It can be useful for eczematous or psoriasiform rashes, constipation, and bloating, as well as kidney and urinary tract disorders.

Second Case Description

A 35-year-old female presented with a 3-year history of facial eruption, which manifested as dryness, redness, and pimple-like lesions. She had no ocular symptoms, and there were no obvious aggravating or ameliorating factors.

Her medical history was significant for anemia, *H. pylori* infection with gastritis and appendicectomy and a heavy menstrual period.

Clinical examination showed erythema, papules with occasional pustules, and underlying edema, especially of the central facial area (Fig. 12.2a). There was no lateralization of symptoms and no aggravating or ameliorating factors noted. From the homeopathic standpoint, the patient had fear of solitude, of unknown and of failure. Strong desire to have last word and love of approval of others was also present. A diagnosis of rosacea was made and the patient placed on homeopathic *Platinum metallicum*, 1 M potency, weekly. At her 6-week follow-up, she had improvement of her facial lesions, only facial erythema present and few papules. This had been preceded by aggravation of her rosacea, following onset of treatment, then amelioration, and then again aggravation, followed by continued amelioration. Her sleep improved and became refreshing. Her anemia was better and her menses remained regular, but no longer with abundant flow. She also claimed to be feeling more "harmony" within herself. Her gastritis improved. All these confirmed that the aggravations were homeopathic, as there was an improvement of her deeper symptoms at the same time as an aggravation of the physical ailment.

She continued to improve and was almost completely lesion-free by her 5-month follow-up (Fig. 12.2b). She continued to remain in remission, with occasional lesions (in stressful situations) up to 15 months after onset of therapy.

A short review of *Platinum metallicum* has been given in the acne section of this chapter. An important distinction to be made is between *Platinum metallicum* and *Aurum metallicum*. Both can be fastidious, can be intolerant of contradiction, and may have fear of failure. However, *Aurum metallicum* is more idealistic than *Platinum metallicum*. *Aurum metallicum* is ambitious in order to do things well, while *Platinum metallicum* often has desire for image behind their ambition. The former is a left-sided medicine and chilly, while the latter is usually a warm and right-sided medicine. Constipation can be a problem for *Aurum metallicum*, who is also very thirsty.

The homeopathic therapy of a case such as this, with rosacea, as well as other ailments—poor sleep, abundant menses, and gastritis with *H. pylori*—would have to be primarily individualized. It would be important to note the order of the appearance of the other physical ailments (this was not possible with this patient). This is because improvement often follows the reverse direction of the appearance of symptoms, with the newest symptoms improving before the older ones. Also, the order of disappearance of the rosacea may also follow the same reverse sequence of appearance. Bearing in

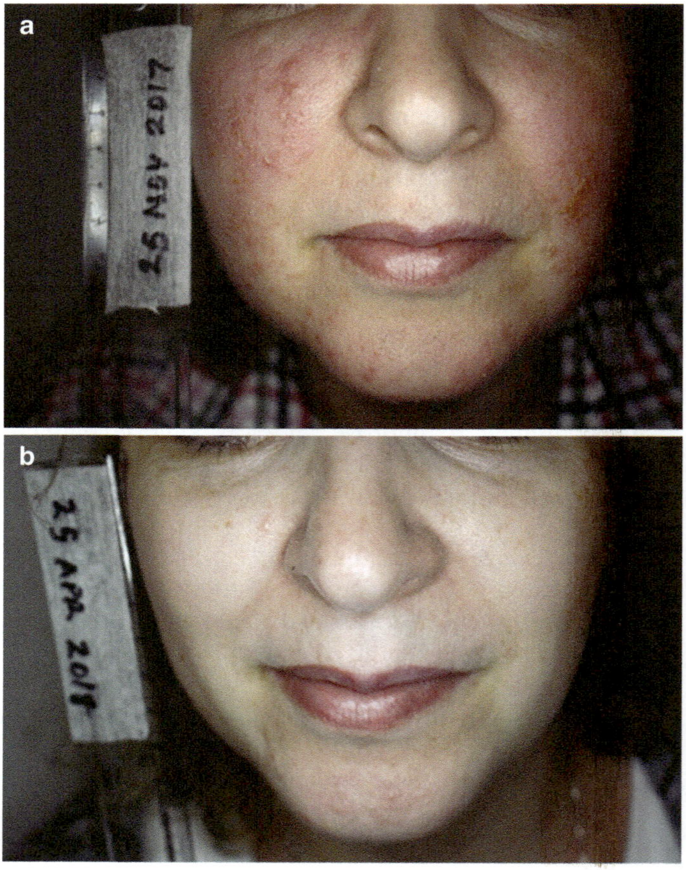

FIGURE 12.2 (**a**) Before onset of treatment, patient with erythematous papules and pustules with edema, in a central facial distribution. (**b**) After 5 months of treatment, lesions completely cleared

mind the comorbidities the patient presented with, it is also possible she would have others, which she may not have noted in her medical history. These may reappear in the course of her healing process transiently. All these issues would need to be discussed with the patient, so she is not alarmed by these phenomena.

Table 12.3 Modified Naranjo criteria for the second case description

Criterion	Points allocated
1	+2
2	+1
3	0
4	+1
5	0
6a	0
6b	0
7	0
8	+1
9	+2
10	+1
Total	8

Supportive homeopathic medications may be required for such issues as poor sleep (e.g., *Coffea cruda*) or abundant menses (*Crotalus horridus*, *Lachesis muta*, *Sepia succus*). These may tide the patient over until the individualized, constitutional medicine takes effect.

Bland dermatocosmetics may be required to help with facial hygiene. This patient received a foundation from a dermatocosmetic brand.

Discussion

Although Dr. S.C. Hahnemann is credited with the founding of homeopathy about 200 years ago, the underlying principle of similars or "like cures like" originates at least from the time of Hippocrates, perhaps even as far back as 1500 B.C. [23]. The principle of similars is a principle whereby the patient is treated with a highly diluted form of medication capable of producing the clinical picture of the disease at a higher concentration, in a healthy human being. The dilutions of medication are known as potencies by homeopaths, and the higher the dilution (potency), the deeper the effect. This means also that lower potencies have more effect on the physical complaints, while higher potencies have a greater tendency to affect the psyche of the patient.

Whichever potency is chosen by the attending physician, it must be the similimum, i.e., the medication picture must be similar to that of the patient's disease picture. As a result, homeopathy is a highly personalized form of treatment.

The mechanism of action of homeopathy is unknown; however, it is known that high dilutions of homeopathy form nanoparticles, using water molecules, that mimic the effects of the original substance [3, 4]. The nanoparticles may then be able to influence physiological functions of the body.

In the treatment of acne, two types of clinical studies were discussed. The first was of a single homeopathic medication trialed on a series of patients. This was based on a "generalized" similimum, using the physical symptoms of acne. There was no placebo control, but the authors of the studies were able to report significantly positive effects of homeopathy on lesion counts, GAGS scores, and Acne-QoL scores [10, 13, 18]. Another study, also using single medications, but on the therapeutic efficacy of acne scars, was done using the medicines *Tuberculinum* and *Sulphur*. This study had placebo control and was able to show an improvement in acne scars following treatment, as compared with the placebo group. Unfortunately, the study did not present the exact medication potencies used for therapy.

The second type of study was a retrospective case series of individualized homeopathic medicines. This comprised 83 patients, with mild, moderate, or severe acne. There was an 81.9% remission rate. The most frequently used medications were homeopathic *Lycopodium clavatum*, *Platinum metallicum*, and *Palladium metallicum* [20]. *Palladium metallicum* was also successfully used in a case presentation, together with *Natrum muriaticum* in a second study [21]. Thus, homeopathy, using either single, disease-specific medications or individualized medicines, might be efficacious in the therapy of acne.

There is less evidence on homeopathic treatment of rosacea. The reasons are not immediately clear. However, a small case presentation ($n = 3$), using individualized homeopathic medicines in erythematotelangiectatic and papulopustular types of rosacea, gave positive results for all three cases. This in itself may be significant, as rosacea can be a very difficult disorder to treat.

Case presentations—one of severe acne and one of severe rosacea—show the effect of homeopathy in difficult-to-treat cases. For the dermatologist, the obvious question, which lies behind their presentation, is "What would I do with such a case, and would I have the same results?" "If so, at what cost by way of side effects and financially?"

Conclusion

Our patients increasingly turn to CAM/integrative medicine for their needs, and we need to be aware of how we can help them. CAM therapies such as herbs, honey, leeches, and light and maggot therapy have already become part of mainstream medicine.

In this regard, homeopathy may become an adjunctive or stand-alone therapy for acne and for rosacea. It can therefore be useful in an integrative setting, especially when patients may feel hesitant about using strong medications such as retinoids, or in situations where cross-reactions with other medications or pregnancy may limit conventional options.

The nature of the individualized approach to homeopathic medicine also suggests that we may need a new paradigm for approaching disease as whole and dermatology in particular. This paradigm would extend to medical research, as the highly holistic, nuanced, and individualized clinical pictures required for therapy in CAM/Integrative medicine do not fit into the framework of double-blind, placebo-controlled trials.

The "placebo effect" may be even more important in CAM/integrative medicine in general, because the consultation itself, when well done, may have a positive impact.

I hope this chapter has shed light on the potential of homeopathy for the therapy of acne and rosacea, thus opening up the possibility for another potential therapeutic option for these disorders.

References

1. Loudon I. A brief history of homeopathy. J R Soc Med. 2006;99(12):607–10. https://doi.org/10.1258/jrsm.99.12.607.
2. Hahnemann SC. Organon der Heilkunst [Organon of the art of medicine]. 6th ed. Lancaster: Gazelle Distribution Trade; 1810.
3. Montagner L, Aïssa J, Ferris S, Montagner J-L, Lavallée C. Electromagnetic signals are produced by aqueous nanostructures derived from bacterial DNA sequences. Interdiscip Sci. 2009;1:81–90.
4. Chickramane PS, Suresh AK, Bellare RJ, Kane GS. Extreme homeopathic dilutions retain starting materials: a nanoparticulate perspective. Homeopathy. 2010;99:231–42.
5. Van Haselen RA. Homeopathic clinical CASE reports: development of a supplement (HOM-CASE) to the CARE clinical case reporting guideline. Complement Ther Med. 2016;25:78–85.
6. Sivamani RK, Morley JE, Rehal B, Armstrong AW. Comparative prevalence of complementary and alternative medicine use among outpatients in dermatology and primary care clinics. JAMA Dermatol. 2014;150(12):1363–5. https://doi.org/10.1001/jamadermatol.2014.2274.
7. Dossett ML, Davis RB, Kaptchuk TJ, Yeh GY. Homeopathy use by US adults: results of a national survey. Am J Public Health. 2016;106(4):743–5. https://doi.org/10.2105/AJPH.2015.303025.
8. Corbin Winslow L, Shapiro H. Physicians want education about complementary and alternative medicine to enhance communication with their patients. Arch Intern Med. 2002;162(10):1176–81. https://doi.org/10.1001/archinte.162.10.1176.
9. Zaenglein AL, Pathy AL, Schlosser BJ, et al. Guidelines of care for the management of acne vulgaris. J Am Acad Dermatol. 2016;74(5):945–73.e33. https://doi.org/10.1016/j.jaad.2015.12.037.

10. Miglani A, Manchanda RK. Prospective, non-randomised, open-label study of homeopathic Z ingiber officinale (ginger) in the treatment of acne vulgaris. Focus Altern Complement Ther. 2014;19:191–7. https://doi.org/10.1111/fct.12140.
11. European Medicines Agency Committee on Herbal Medicinal Products (HMPC). Assessment report on Zingiber officinale Roscoe, rhizoma. [Online] Available at: https://www.ema.europa.eu/en/documents/herbal-report/draft-assessment-report-zingiberis-rhizoma_en.pdf.
12. Allen TF. Zingiber. In: The encyclopedia of pure materia medica, vol. 10. New York: Boericke and Tafel; 1879. p. 225. Available at: https://collections.nlm.nih.gov/bookviewer?PID=nlm:nlmuid-64240040RX10-mvpart#page/8/mode/2up.
13. Miglani A, Manchanda RK. Observational study of Arctium lappa in the treatment of acne vulgaris. Homeopathy. 2014;103(3):203–7. https://doi.org/10.1016/j.homp.2013.12.002.
14. Chan YS, Cheng LN, Wu JH, Chan E, Kwan YW, Lee SM, et al. A review of the pharmacological effects of Arctium lappa (burdock). Inflammopharmacology. 2011;19:245–54. https://doi.org/10.1007/s10787-010-0062-4.
15. Committee on Herbal Medicinal Products (HMPC). Herbal monograph. [Online] Available at: https://www.ema.europa.eu/en/documents/herbal-monograph/final-community-herbal-monograph-arctium-lappa-l-radix_en.pdf.
16. Murphy R. Lappa Arctium. In: Nature's materia medica. Blacksburg: Lotus Health Institute; 2006.
17. Alzohairy MA. Therapeutics role of Azadirachta indica (Neem) and their active constituents in diseases prevention and treatment. Evid Based Complement Alternat Med. 2016;2016:7382506. https://doi.org/10.1155/2016/7382506.
18. Miglani A, Manchanda RK. Azadirachta indica in treatment of acne vulgaris – an open-label observational study. Indian J Res Homeopath. 2014;8:218–23.
19. Shraddhamayananda S. An observation on successful treatment of acne scar with homeopathic medicine. Int J Biopharm. 2015;6(1):27–31.
20. Nwabudike LC. Homeopathy in the treatment of acne. E-poster P00051, 25th European Academy of Dermatology and Venereology Conference. Vienna; 2016.

21. Nwabudike LC. Case reports of acne and homeopathy. Complement Med Res. 2018;25:52–5. https://doi.org/10.1159/000486309.
22. Nwabudike LC. Rosacea and homeopathy. Proc Rom Acad Ser B. 2012;14(3):207–11.
23. Bellavite P, Conforti A, Piasere V, Ortolani R. Immunology and homeopathy. 1. Historical background. Evid Based Complement Alternat Med. 2005;2(4):441–52. https://doi.org/10.1093/ecam/neh141.

Index

R. N. Rupani, P. A. Lio (eds.), *Integrative Dermatology*,
https://doi.org/10.1007/978-3-030-58954-7

GPSR Compliance

The European Union's (EU) General Product Safety Regulation (GPSR) is a set of rules that requires consumer products to be safe and our obligations to ensure this.

If you have any concerns about our products, you can contact us on ProductSafety@springernature.com

In case Publisher is established outside the EU, the EU authorized representative is:

Springer Nature Customer Service Center GmbH
Europaplatz 3
69115 Heidelberg, Germany

Batch number: 10732632

Printed by Printforce, the Netherlands